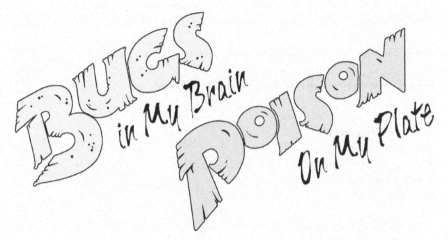

Bugs in My Brain, Poison On My Plate

Using M-Field Energy Signature Matching to Optimize Your Health

Dr. Frank Springob with
Sydney Upham Soelter, M.A.

BALBOA.
PRESS

A DIVISION OF HAY HOUSE

Interior Graphics/Art Credit: Matt House, James Taylor and James Dowlen

Balboa Press books may be ordered through booksellers or by contacting:

Balboa Press
A Division of Hay House
1663 Liberty Drive
Bloomington, IN 47403
www.balboapress.com
1-(877) 407-4847

ISBN: 978-1-4525-5646-8 (sc)
ISBN: 978-1-4525-5648-2 (hc)
ISBN: 978-1-4525-5647-5 (e)

Library of Congress Control Number: 2012914468

Printed in the United States of America

Balboa Press rev. date: 08/14/2012

Dedication

To Linda, my life partner, mother of my children, nutrition therapist and Wellness Center manager—and to all of the other courageous healers battling the perversion of our food and the suppression of the truth.

To our children, grandchildren, and all future children, that they may always have unadulterated food to eat, as the Supreme Power originally intended.

To Autumn, co-creator of MFT.

"The Field is the thing."

Albert Einstein

Contents

Foreword

It is a pleasure and an honor to be asked to write the foreword to Frank's new book. I have known Dr. Springob since we first became acquainted in chiropractic school in the early 1970's. He has been a true friend and colleague in the healing arts.

Frank has dedicated himself to helping mankind through his keen observation of the human condition. He has dedicated his life's work to natural health care and he does this through his affable use of insight, humor and intuition. This book portrays his life's journey in his latest evolution in energetic medicine.

He walks you through his life experiences to gain insight into his discoveries, both observed and experienced, derived from his many years of providing care. His questions and concerns all relate to his efforts to improve the quality of the human experience. Frank takes nothing for granted and the result is a book which is sure to lead you on the path to an improved expression of personal health.

This endeavor comes at a risk which he acknowledges and yet he is willing to undertake. New discoveries are first scoffed at, gradually accepted and then become incorporated into a known body of information. Frank presents a new perspective for those who are ready to begin an adventure in their own quest for health. Your personal quest for health and well-being is certainly a lifetime journey that must be earned and re-won every day.

Great innovators challenge us through their concepts to look at the available information and to draw our own conclusions about its application and potential benefit to one's own life. Frank does nothing more than that and this latest information comes to the reader through the personal interpretation of their own Innate Intelligence. The healing power in all of us is provided by our Creator.

Frank sees the big picture and shares with you his rendition of the ideal nutritional realm in hopes that you will be able to paint your life's canvas with brilliance and majesty; that is our ultimate destiny. Where you were is but a thought; where you are now is the beginning of a destiny of free will. Through better health, I join Frank in the hope that you will be able to fully express that majestic piece of God that is within all of us.

Meed A. West, D.C., N.D., F.A.C.O.

Introduction

In my 36 year history of clinical practice in the natural healing arts, I have had more than 300,000 individual patient encounters. Along the way, I have read hundreds of books and attended more than 150 professional seminars. In the early years, I was attracted to educational materials that improved my diagnostic abilities, wishing to advance my patient's overall health as efficiently as possible.

I was encouraged by those patients who made progress under my care, but those who did not were the ones I focused upon. I was unrelenting in my quest for answers to the unknown variables that blocked improvement. So, although I live in an isolated area, I made frequent weekend trips to Seattle or Portland to attend post-graduate educational seminars. It was a quest for the "magic bullet", the one treatment or procedure that would make natural healing complete.

My personal history of severe headaches in my youth and the relief I received through chiropractic care was a strong motivator in this mission; it was the one treatment that had given me relief. When I began my practice in the mid-1970s, I was positive that I could "fix" anyone's headaches. Unfortunately, it turned out not to be true. There were many headache cases that responded well, but some that did not.

The true reality was difficult for me. I helped hundreds of people, but the *hidden key* to the resolution of many cases still eluded me. I would get glimpses of truth in some of the new learned procedures that would assist in certain situations, such as improvement in premenstrual headaches after supplementation with vitamin B6. I had read that vitamin B6 helped modulate the estrogen levels which were higher in the body just before a woman started her cycle. In practice, the introduction of B6 not only helped with the premenstrual headaches, some of these patients also reported dramatic relief from water retention and a higher level of mental well-being. Then, after a few cycles, it would quit working. I was left asking myself, what is still missing?

This idea of nutritional deficiencies being the missing link interested me. I had always had the core belief that the food created by God would give us the nutrients we need. In chiropractic school, we were told, "The Power that made the body is the Power that heals the body." Well, the Power that made the body also made the food. Therefore, the *food* should assist in that healing.

It raised questions about the ability of our current food supply to fully nourish the body. It was not a matter of food quantity; it was a matter of food quality.

Why were people having health problems that were improved by *components* of food, such as B6 for PMS? Since menstruation is a normal female variant, why should there be symptoms associated with the monthly cycle that can be relieved with a supplement? That component should have already been in the food, and supplementation should not be necessary. Yet, it was... and it did not always work. What was I missing?

One possible conclusion was that God forgot something in the food. A more probable conclusion, and the one I came to believe, was that we humans who processed the food "messed it up" somehow.

The idea of "junk food" was first introduced to me while still a student. *Prevention* and *Organic Gardening* magazines were fixtures in the apartment I shared with my chiropractic school roommates, Bob Ernst and Meed West. Bob was a huge fan of J.I. Rodale, the late founder and publisher of those two periodicals.

One night in 1971, I had planned to watch The Dick Cavett Show, when J.I. Rodale was the guest to be interviewed. As Dick Cavett recalled, Mr. Rodale was the first guest interviewed that night. During the interview, the 72 year old Mr. Rodale stated that he planned to live to be 100 years old, unless he was run over by a hypoglycemic cab driver. Moments later, Mr. Rodale, the icon for healthful living, slumped over and died during the taping. That show never aired.

Reading this in the newspaper the next day was a defining moment in my life. I had many conflicting thoughts about that event which I spent years sorting out in my mind. The first thought was, "If eating right is so important, why did J.I. Rodale die on television?" He was, after all, the poster boy for perfect health. Although I did not completely reject the concept regarding the importance of proper diet, I certainly was not convinced.

Additional conflicting thoughts occurred when J.I.'s son, Robert Rodale, took over as publisher of *Prevention* magazine. Suddenly, there were advertisements appearing that were not present when his father was at the helm . . . ads for over-the-counter pain killers and other products from the pharmaceutical industry. I was led to question the new publisher's integrity and commitment to the concepts of natural healing. I saw this change in the advertising policy as "selling out", a phrase we used a lot in those days.

I was searching for natural healing theories so true and immutable, that nobody would even consider selling out as an option. I wanted precepts that were so clear and obvious that denying them would be like Peter denying Jesus. What were those truths?

All of the questioning and searching eventually led me to a new paradigm of natural healthcare. This book is about the evolution of experience and thought that ultimately gave birth to a new method of nutritional and energy healing. This is the story of the creation of *M-Field Signature Matching* and a structured process of testing for nutritional energy signature compatibility.

The M-Field is your body's unique *energy signature*, named after the Morphinogenic Field or Morphogenic Field recognized by Dr. Albert Einstein and Dr. Royal Lee in their separate groundbreaking research projects in the first half of the 20th Century. The entire testing procedure is called the Morphogenic Field Technique® (MFT).

The initial steps of the MFT Testing Procedure are designed to find nutritional deficiencies and toxicities. Once these are uncovered, the final step is to match the *energy signatures* of the food and the whole food supplements to the *energy signature* of the individual being tested. This step is called M-Field Signature Matchingsm.

For those who have a background in *energy thinking*, these ideas will not be new. People who have studied the basics of quantum physics will be familiar with the theories, but the practical application of the concepts at the nutrient-level might be new. Those who have training or experience in energy healing may even find this healing technique to be simplistic. To others, it will seem odd and possibly unbelievable.

Practitioners of allopathic medicine have typically tended to reject anything that has its origins from outside the pharmaceutical industry or political medicine. Including my time as a student, I have been involved in the chiropractic profession for 40 years. The closed-minded nature of political medicine has never ceased to amaze me. The AMA and its allies have spent the better part of 100 years trying to eliminate the perceived competition from the natural healing professions such as chiropractic, naturopathy and acupuncture.

35 years ago there was an anti-trust lawsuit filed against the AMA and others to stop the blatant attacks. Chiropractic was the clear winner of the lawsuit, yet the discrimination continues to this day. While the tactics have changed a bit, the intent remains clear: suppress any information that is threatening to the medical monopoly.

It requires an open mind to appreciate the potential of M-Field Signature Matching. It is natural to question new ideas, especially when they take you far away from the status quo of the contemporary health care paradigm. Albert Einstein once expressed that there were fewer than five people in the whole world who truly understood the physics theory of relativity. It is now accepted science. Any new idea will have its skeptics, and rightfully so. We would be foolish to not challenge new thinking. However, we would be equally foolish to reject bold new ideas without consideration, simply because they are unfamiliar.

This book offers a new, truly-natural healing alternative to the mindless default of prescribing a drug for every problem. It rejects the notion that anyone can create health by adding a man-made chemical to the body. While symptoms can be altered and crises can be managed with drugs, real health is achieved by giving the body the nutrients it needs to repair the damage done by our increasingly artificial world. If you are trying to build health, you don't need one more chemical! You do need the real, whole food that will actually nourish the body.

Every person is one of a kind, with nutritional needs that are as unique as they are. While nutritional systems that are aimed at everyone may offer something that some people will benefit from, it is impossible for a mass-marketed product to address the unique specific nutritional needs of every individual who buys it.

The Morphogenic Field Technique addresses <u>individual</u> needs only. It is not a canned, planned program like most of the so-called nutritional products seen advertised on television. Commercials for those systems are aimed at *everyone*, which means they are not exactly right for *anyone*. With MFT and M-Field Signature Matching, we can be "exactly right" for each person we test.

We don't make claims about treating any condition, diagnosis or other label. We only make one claim: we will expand and balance your energy field using our procedure. When performed on a systematic basis, the M-Field grows, becomes symmetrical, and there is corresponding natural health improvement. The entire MFT testing procedure can be performed by a skilled practitioner in 3 to 5 minutes. Compared to other health care procedures it is relatively inexpensive and noninvasive, and helps people to know precisely what their body needs for optimum health.

Through this book, I will tell two parallel stories. The first is of the development of the M-Field Technique, including the work of the health care pioneers who risked ridicule to advance their science. The second story tells the tale of the degradation of our food sources for power and profit, emphasizing my concern for the health of our children and grandchildren. At the end, practical solutions are proposed for reversing food degradation and creating lasting health. My wish is for us all to feel the hope of a future where food once again *feeds* us, a future that can be ours if we take back our food supply.

As a dedicated natural health care professional, I know that I am in good company. The MFT procedure has been a tremendous gift to me and my colleague and co-creator, Autumn Smith, NTP, and the rest of the staff here at Boulevard Natural Wellness Clinic. Since making the discovery three years ago, we have taught the MFT procedure at professional seminars throughout the Pacific Northwest. These seminars have been well attended, and the feedback we have received confirms that these skills, although developed at our Wellness Center in Port Angeles, are highly transferrable to others. It has been my privilege to develop this technique and to share this gift with my patients, my colleagues, and now, my readers.

I hope you enjoy the stories.

Frank Springob, Summer 2012
Port Angeles, Washington

Chapter 1

The Science of Energy and Nutritional Healing

"A fact is a simple statement that everyone believes. It is innocent, unless found guilty. A hypothesis is a novel suggestion that no one wants to believe. It is guilty, until found effective."

-Edward Teller

My attraction to science was inherent. From my youth, I was intrigued by the idea of drawing conclusions from observation and experience. I was particularly interested in the realm of physics, although I didn't use that word in those days. Although I am not a physicist, my perspective in my chosen profession of chiropractic has been based upon the laws of physics; first *Newtonian*, and now *Quantum*.

Physics can be broken down into very simple ideas based upon the *scale or size* of the matter in question. Simply put, it is not about the matter of physics; it is about the physics of matter. Great big things have a different physics than very small things.

When thinking of great big things, we can imagine our own solar system. The basic physics of the dynamic workings in our solar system is gravity, which is the foundation of *Gravitational Physics*. Very large objects have a gravitational attraction to other very large objects in their *gravitational neighborhood*. When it comes to a solar system, the neighborhood is not "down the block and around the corner." The next door neighbor in our solar system can be tens of millions of miles away.

1

Our home, the Earth, is routinely affected by the closest *house next door*, the moon. The push and pull effect of the moon's gravity is the factor that controls the ocean tides. Of course, we cannot *see* gravity as it does its work. In order to experience the effect, you must go to the beach and watch the change of the tides.

This demonstrates the basic problem with most energy healing---up until now, we have not had a way to measure or quantify it. In the world of science, nothing has validity until it can be measured. This can be a double edged sword. For a person of science, having objective evidence is the only acceptable way to approach any subject in a rational manner. Unfortunately, this doesn't give acknowledgement to the vast number of people who *know what they feel*. The people who are experienced in energy healing have a "sense" of the energy that most people cannot relate to.

In Health Care, we live in an age of objective accountability, of "evidence-based" outcomes. Health Care professionals are no longer able to treat patients unless they can measure the results of their efforts, especially if they expect a third party payor to cover it. Employers and employees alike are spending ever-increasing amounts of money to pay health insurance premiums. Although it is not unusual for patients to have health problems that are unresolved by contemporary medicine, when patients seek alternative care, insurance companies often refuse to reimburse them, saying that there is no evidence of its effectiveness.

Surprisingly, alternative care is held to a higher standard of outcome measurement than mainstream medical care. The rules for insurance reimbursement are selectively enforced. By proclaiming alternative procedures "medically unnecessary", insurance companies effectively switch the burden of proof to the alternative provider. The third party payor does not have to pay for the treatment if the provider has difficulty measuring the outcome. The patient's subjective report of improvement is not sufficient to justify third-party payment.

In order to prove the scientific validity of our energy healing technique, it must be based upon established science. An explanation of the physics involved helps to illustrate the science behind the MFT energy signature matching. Examining the physics of the big things, such as planets, can help us understand the physics of little things, like the subatomic particles that are responsible for the M-Field.

Most of us living on the planet are aware of the physical phenomenon we call gravity. Students learn in elementary school that the larger the planet, the greater the *gravitational field*. A person standing on Jupiter would weigh more than a person standing on Earth. A person standing on the earth would weigh more than a person standing on the moon. This became much easier to comprehend once we had video of humans doing physical activities on the moon. The *seeing* became *believing*.

Further down the scale, on the surface of the planet, the gravitational attraction of objects such as people, buildings, and vehicles is considered *negligible*. It still exists, but we don't find ourselves being sucked into a building just because it is much bigger than we are. The physics theory that applies to objects of this size is called *Newtonian Physics*.

Gravitational Physics describes objects the size of planets, and *Newtonian Physics* describes things the size of people, cars and buildings. On an even smaller scale, the system that applies to the atoms, molecules and subatomic particles of body chemistry is called *Quantum Physics*. It is the physics of the little pieces, and similar to gravity, it cannot be seen.

When Albert Einstein discussed these forces that act between elementary particles in the early 20th Century, nobody understood it. To many people, quantum physics is still not "real" because we do not encounter it on a day-to-day basis in any way that requires us to consciously think about it. Although we employ quantum physics every day when turning on a light switch, using a computer or watching television, these actions do not require that we understand what is happening on a subatomic level.

Quantum Physics is about *the energy that holds it all together*. This is the same energy we use in MFT to develop nutritional protocols and discover toxic body energies.

The human body is made up of many organ systems, such as the nervous, digestive, reproductive, and circulatory systems. Each organ system is made up of individual organs. For example, the digestive system includes the oral cavity, the esophagus, the stomach, the pancreas, liver, gall bladder, the small and large intestine, to name a few.

Each organ can contain a variety of tissue types, including connective tissue, epithelial tissue, muscle tissue or nerve tissue. Each form of tissue is made up of multiple cells, and each cell is made up of multiple organelles such as the cell nucleus, membrane and mitochondria. Within these tiny microcosms, there are thousands of energetic and chemical processes going on each minute, all the time. Ultimately, as we go smaller and smaller, we get to what is really at the core----<u>ENERGY!</u>

Everything in the universe, fundamentally, is energy; it all emits an *energy signature*. Physics research papers try to bring the energy signature alive for the reader by drawing illustrations of the theoretical concept. Over the last hundred years, many books have been written that discuss the human body from an energy perspective, although not many have been best-sellers. Most of the literature on the subject is considered unconventional, outside of the mainstream. MFT brings a new concept to the discussion of the practical application of energy theory: namely, matching the energy signature of the person with the energy signatures of food for optimal health.

As the health care crisis in this country has escalated, there is an equivalent food crisis that has escalated in parallel. The dramatic increase in artificial and synthetic components added to our food has changed the very nature of our diet. Many of us grew up in the age of "Better Living through Chemistry", the slogan of the chemical industry. Now, non-food additives have become so commonplace that we have become anesthetized to the psychological impact of eating chemical substances named "sucrose acetate isobutyrate", "glyceryl abietate", or "polyethylene glycol", to name just a few.

In the 21st Century, we have a situation that requires special words to describe the origin of our food. Real food is now called "organic" food, while fake food, or food that has been altered to the point where it now has very little nutrition, is called "commercial" food, or just "food".

When we changed our food, we put our very survival at risk. When the energy signature of the food is incompatible with the energy signature of the body, the body will not recognize that food as something nourishing. It will look upon the food as an invader and attack it! Herein lays the problem with imposter foods such as Olestra and aspartame. Manufactured with the intention of "tricking" the body into not absorbing it as calories, these artificial substances provoke an immune response. Rather than building up the body, the fake foods tear it down, draining it of resources and stamina.

The end result is predictable: more disease, more autoimmune challenges and more cancer will be our future. We have already seen it happening, yet most of us feel powerless to do anything about it. Stemming the tide of the poisoned-plate onslaught begins with education. We must stand up against the forces that are destroying our food supply! All great things that have ever been accomplished in this country began when the people took a stand for what is right!

The American Revolution came about because loyal Colonists grew tired of British suppression and eventually were forced to act. A similar situation is building in America today. Our food supply is in the control of a few mega-corporations with aggressive marketing campaigns designed to suppress the truth and ensure their own profits. Such a corrupt system, based upon disinformation and greed, should not be allowed to exist in this country.

Much of this food is readily available and cheap because of government subsidies, particularly to the corn industry, which received an astounding $80,609,075,462 in subsidies in the years 1995-2010, according to the 2011 Farm Subsidy Database. *Eighty billion dollars to keep corn syrup cheap for companies such as Coca-Cola and Kellogg's!* Something is wrong with this picture. We were once the *Land of the Free*, but when it comes to our food, we are free no longer. We live in the *Land of the **Controlled and Manipulated**.* It is time for a new revolution, one without violence or anarchy, as we reclaim our rightful heritage to not merely stay alive, but thrive on the bounty of our planet.

Chapter 2

Conundrum

"If people let government decide what foods they eat and what medicines they take, their bodies will soon be in as sorry a state as are the souls of those who live under tyranny."

-Thomas Jefferson

We live in interesting times. The United States of America is considered the richest nation on Earth, yet we are also the greatest debtor nation that the world has ever seen, with a national debt of over 13 trillion dollars. With a culture and lifestyle that is envied around the world, the USA represents a land of plenty.

The American health care system is extremely technologically advanced. We have diagnostic procedures for every acute health complaint. If you must have a medical emergency, there is no better place to be than at the modern American hospital emergency room. Yet, according to the World Health Organization, we have a serious flaw in our system: the United States ranks 37th, out of 38, in total health for industrialized countries. We outspend everyone looking for health, but real health still eludes us.

We have many other serious problems in addition to our economy and our environment. Over the past four decades, the ecological movement has challenged us all to use resources and raw materials sustainably. We hear concerns on a global scale about the availability of a fresh water supply. As the population of the earth continues to grow, how can we care for our limited resources?

The recent American financial crisis has required a hard look at our country's habit of spending more than is collected in revenue. There have been accusations of irresponsible government spending at both the state and federal levels. Instead of a sustainable long-term response, we just keep kicking the financial can down the road. This has occurred on a personal level for many Americans as well. We live in an instant gratification society; we want **what** we want, **when** we want it. Acting on these impulses creates credit card debt and home mortgages that collapse upon the borrower.

More and more, the question of sustainability is raised in any discussion of future endeavors. Whether regarding health care, economics, ecology, or agriculture, this is a question that ultimately must be answered.

Unsustainable

People who are familiar with pop music from the 60's may recall a popular song by folk artist Barry Maguire:

> "The eastern world, it is exploding.
> Violence flaring, bullets loading.
> You're old enough to kill, but not for voting.
> And even the Jordan River has bodies floating.
> You don't believe in war, but what's that gun you're toting?
> And you tell me, over and over and over and over again,
> That you don't believe we're on the eve of destruction."

This song, titled "The Eve of Destruction", spent several weeks at the top of the charts and fit within the genre of the protest songs in style at that time. It questioned the logic and sustainability of the military industrial complex controlling the political conversation in a world of stockpiled nuclear weapons.

When it comes to food, America has reached "The Nutritional Eve of Destruction". How much longer can we continue the farming practices that have been perverted by large corporate conglomerates? Big agribusiness has bought up family farms, poisoned the soil with pesticides and herbicides, and then genetically modified the seeds to grow better on the poisoned soil. Monsanto and other large companies have genetically modified the seeds to make them sterile, and then patented the seeds, thus requiring farmers to purchase new seeds each year.

Gone are the days of the "Circle of Life" on the farm. Done in the name of efficiency, this leaves both farmers and consumers at the mercy of the corporations that now own the "rights" to our food. Big Agribusiness has also manipulated the political system to infiltrate the regulatory agencies with their own people. These "plants" are then perfectly positioned to write policies that benefit the corporations at the expense of the consumer...the consumer whom these agencies exist to protect. While their spokespeople spin the conversation to make it sound as if these corporations have the best interest of the consumer in mind, the real motives are clear: control the food supply to ensure present and future profit.

Barry Maguire obviously hit a nerve with his haunting lyrics that resonated with his strong message, especially when combined with a driving militaristic musical arrangement. "The Eve of Destruction" sold millions of records and was a rallying cry for much of the political change that followed over the next decade. Of course, not everyone agreed with that message. Many military leaders and defense contractors saw nothing wrong with this course of action. The people who lived through those times were caught up in a huge political tug-of-war about the direction this country should take. Under John F. Kennedy's leadership, the country had just survived the Cuban Missile Crisis and was confronted with the challenge of the spread of communism. Later, with JFK gone, there was new leadership and a different agenda.

Much of the generation that had lived through World War II considered the political protests of the 1960's to be unpatriotic and anti-American. Their rallying cry was, "America, Love It or Leave It." Those of the younger generation protested, considering the actions of the United States military to be criminal in nature. Their slogan of unity was, "America, Change It or Lose It." It was an epic battle of two very diverse ideologies, waged under a subtle, yet constant, nuclear threat.

Now, four decades later, we face a new silent threat! While it is not as obvious as the peril of impending nuclear war, it is very real and it threatens our survival just the same. The nutrient content of our food is diminishing to the point where soon, it may no longer support life. Powerful pesticides and herbicides leach from the soil into our mainstream food sources, and eventually into livestock and wildlife. Ultimately, these poisons will overwhelm the immune system of every animal in the food chain.

This threat has crept up on us slowly over the past 150 years, but has recently accelerated as big agribusiness has become more aggressive in their efforts to control the food. Unfortunately, subtle changes over a long time frame do not create glaring, hard to ignore headlines. Unlike Vietnam, it does not require a military draft that disrupts the lives of our young people. We are like the proverbial "Frog in Boiling Water", living in an instant gratification society where it is easy to sit back and wait until the problem becomes so painful we can no longer ignore it. When it comes to the food we depend upon to nourish and renew our bodies, we cannot wait until the heat becomes unbearable . . . if we do, it will be too late.

Evolution

As a practicing Natural Health Care Professional (HCP) in Port Angeles, Washington for the past 36 years, I have witnessed a slow but consistent deterioration in both the diet and the health of the patients that I treat. Like many other HCP's, I have utilized a form of nutritional analysis called "muscle response testing" throughout my career.

Over these four decades, the science of muscle response testing has evolved. First developed by Dr. George Goodheart, it is essentially a form of communication with the human body. Muscle response testing originated within the chiropractic profession, where it was first used for the purpose of simultaneously correcting both nutritional and structural health problems.

I have witnessed several incarnations and refinements to this infant science, and have followed these improvements with great interest. In fact, I have attended most of the available seminars offered in the professional world on the subject. Study and clinical practice have convinced me that the best way to get up-to-date nutritional information from the body is by using a properly performed muscle response test. To use a computer term, it is now possible to "download" a great deal of analytical information about the current state of the patient's health using structured muscle response testing techniques.

Forty years removed from my first muscle response test, my reality was radically changed by a simple statement. It came from Autumn Renee Smith, a then-21-year-old Nutritional Therapy student who was working in our Wellness Center one late spring afternoon. It was an ingenious statement; so obvious once she said it, yet it was something that I had never considered! It was the type of statement that can only come from "fresh eyes."

In her training, Autumn had learned that the cell was the basic unit of body structure: the cells combine to make the tissues, which cumulatively create the internal organs. Aware that the function of the muscle response test was to focus on the energy emitted from various organs and glands, Autumn mused, "I do not understand why we test the organs. Wouldn't it be better to talk to the cells? If we could, we would catch these problems earlier in the nutritional healing process."

In that moment, I did not have an answer. It was a simple, yet brilliant, question. Despite my vast clinical experience with muscle response testing, I had never thought of it.

Autumn's inspired observation set us on a new path of nutritional healing. We embarked upon the next evolution in the established science of muscle response testing, a new journey of *energy signature testing* of our food supply. Through this discovery, practitioners and patients can now immediately identify what the body needs and does not need for optimum health and wellness.

We called our new science the Morphogenic Field Technique® (MFT). It utilizes up-to-date, established quantum physics science and combines it with the classic concept of feeding the body organic whole food nutrition. The potential to improve the overall health of a person is based upon the ability to match the energy of the individual with the energy of their food or food supplements. In Morphogenic Field Technique, we have nicknamed the procedure, "the quantum conversation," between the body and the food.

Innate Intelligence

Within the philosophical origins of the chiropractic profession, there exists the concept of *Innate Intelligence*. Simply stated, this is the built-in ability for the body to heal itself, given the right environment. "Innate Intelligence" refers to the body's ability to heal, once the *subluxation* or mechanical spinal blockage to the nervous system is removed. Innate Intelligence is spoken of in chiropractic school, not as a concept, but as an entity unto itself. In the profession, the word "Innate" can be used interchangeably with words like "God Force" or "Life Force".

The words *Innate Intelligence* have found their way into other professions and philosophies as well, as the nervous system and its related energy fields have broad applications in other health disciplines. Some scientists like to use the phrase "intelligent design", which sounds similar, for the same purpose. It can also be used interchangeably with other nebulous phrases such as "healing ability" or "Source Energy."

As described by D.D. Palmer, the Founder of the Chiropractic Profession, *vertebral subluxation* is a blockage to the Innate's ability to provide the body with the energy needed for constant, unobstructed healing. The story of the first chiropractic adjustment given in Davenport, Iowa on September 18, 1895 clearly illustrates this line of thought.

As the story goes, a janitor named Harvey Lillard had suffered from hearing loss for the better part of two decades. Dr. Palmer had the intention of helping this patient by releasing the flow of nervous system energy that was mechanically blocked, inhibiting auditory function. Based upon the case history given by Mr. Lillard, Dr. Palmer reasoned that a distortion (subluxation) in the patient's neck may be responsible for the dysfunction.

Dr. Palmer, after analyzing the nature of the distortion, delivered the very first chiropractic adjustment and Mr. Lillard's hearing was subsequently restored. The chiropractic profession was born! Dr. Palmer's intention to improve the life of another human being resulted in the creation of what is now the largest natural healing profession in the world. The chiropractic mission became the correction of vertebral subluxation to allow the normal function of Innate Intelligence, the body's natural healing energy.

Intention Multiplied

Although he could not possibly have realized it at that time, millions of lives have been changed and improved as a result of this simple intention. As one of thousands of graduates of Palmer College of Chiropractic, I have experienced the long-term result of Dr. Palmer's intention on a deeply personal level.

In my 36 years of clinical practice, I have delivered somewhere between two and three million individual "segmental" chiropractic adjustments. Although few of these adjustments have produced the dramatic results achieved by D.D. Palmer with Mr. Lilliard, I have seen my share of clinical miracles as well.

In our Wellness Center in Port Angeles, we have the good fortune to hear these fantastic stories of healing from our chiropractic patients and nutritional therapy clients on a daily basis. Some of our success stories develop from chiropractic, finding and correcting nerve pressure of mechanical origin. Once the pressure is relieved, the Innate Intelligence is allowed to flow again. More recently, with the advent of the MFT Procedure, many of our success stories relate to the use of the energy field of the body to find nutritional deficiencies and toxic overload in our patients. Removing these "nutritional subluxations" creates great healing, and thereby creates great healing stories.

Bugs in My Brain

You will find some of these healing stories woven throughout this book. Each one is written by the patient who lived the experience. The first, Chantea's Story, is one of my favorites and a classic example of the power of the MFT Procedure. We were able to address Chantea's symptoms from a perspective that could not and would not be used in the world of traditional American medicine. The MFT Test Kits identified the *energy of parasites* in her small intestine, heart and brain. Her astonishment was evident in her remark, "You mean I have **bugs in my brain??**"

When I say the "energy of parasites", this is exactly what I mean. The MFT Procedure *finds* the energy and the MFT Protocol *treats* the energy. MFT Practitioners do not, in the strict sense, treat the parasite. The hardest concept for most patients to understand is that we do not treat a microbe; we treat the *energy* of a microbe. However, even the most skeptical patients are soon convinced, as they are liberated from their symptoms and begin to experience the wellbeing that comes with effective, natural healing.

Chantea's parasite energy was treated with a completely natural approach. It was affordable, effective, and completely free of unwanted side effects.

The solution to all of our MFT Procedure findings is a protocol that is nutritional, herbal, or sometimes homeopathic, but always truly natural.

Poison on My Plate

What you put into your mouth in the present is the most important factor affecting your health in the future. While there are many variables to health and disease, the old adage, "You are what you eat", has never been more fitting. The quality of our food supply has been under unrelenting attack for decades. This is not a new story; it has been told over and over again. In the 1930's, Dr. Royal Lee wrote and lectured extensively on sickness resulting from poisoning by commercial food. Unfortunately, little has been accomplished to reverse the trend of this degradation, and now we all sit at our tables with a super-sized portion of "Poison on our Plates."

Chapter 3

The "M-Field"

"Everything should be made as simple as possible, but not simpler."

~Albert Einstein

What is the nature of this field? The Morphogenic Field, or M-Field, is a manifestation of the same life-force energy that Dr. Palmer had the intention of releasing in Harvey Lilliard. Although it cannot be seen, the M-field is a part of the nervous system of every human being. For all of us, everyday bodily functions produce subtle electrical currents, some of which can be measured with technology, such as an electrocardiograph tracking the electrical energy of the heart. Many basic biochemical reactions, from thoughts to digestion, involve the shuffling of charged particles. All of this activity contributes to the energy field surrounding the body.

It is a well-known fact that every electrical field is accompanied by an electromagnetic field that surrounds it and shadows its level of intensity. A large, intense electromagnetic field (EMF) is emitted by high-voltage electrical lines, while the wiring in a house creates a relatively small EMF. Most of us have had the experience of driving in a car with the radio on. The radio reception is normal until the car approaches high-voltage power lines overhead. Suddenly, your nice clear radio signal becomes a wall of static when the high-voltage electrical current flowing through the power lines interferes. The power lines emit a surrounding electromagnetic field, which scramble the signal from the radio station. As the car moves away from the power lines, the signal once again becomes clear.

The nervous system, including the brain, the spinal cord and the peripheral nerves in your arms and legs, also gives off a surrounding field of electromagnetic energy. This energy field is acknowledged in other cultures. Known as "chi" or "life force", it is the foundation of some of the ancient healing arts and a few forms of martial arts. Similar to the EMF's surrounding power lines, the M-Field is an extension of the energy of the body's nervous system.

The Torus Energy Pattern

The M-Field can be visualized as an outline of energy commonly referred to in the scientific realm as the "Torus Energy Pattern". As you can see from the illustrations, this common pattern can be found within the universe as a primary configuration at all levels. From the smallest atomic particles, to the cross section of an apple, the energy field of the human, the electromagnetic field of the earth, or the shape of the galaxy, the repetition of the torus leads us to the conclusion that it represents a basic arrangement in the geometry of life.

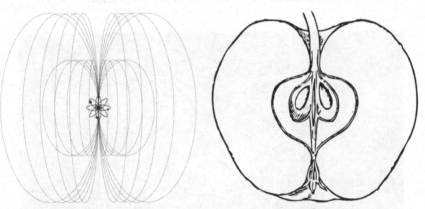

At the quantum scale, a side by side comparison of atomic torus and the apple show the consistency of the pattern.

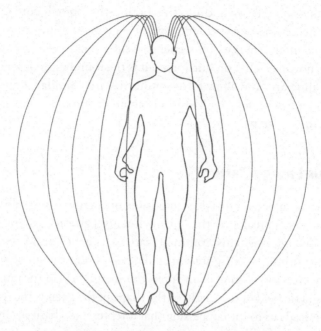

The M-Field surrounding the human demonstrates the uniformity
of the torus pattern on the Newtonian scale.

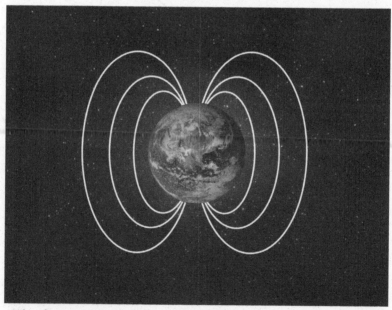

The electromagnetic field of the Earth and other planets form the
torus pattern on the gravitational scale.

While each scale of matter (gravitational, Newtonian, and quantum) has different physical laws, the torus pattern is a constant within all levels of physics. Scientific research has been attempting to unify the rules of physics for decades. At least 15 different variations of "String Theory" have been proposed during this quest, but none have met the challenge of explaining the variations in the laws of physics as we know them. However, it appears that the torus pattern, known since the early 20th Century, is one constant at all levels, and so holds promise for greater understanding of physics.

It is our contention that the human torus energy pattern, the M-Field, is the origin of the body's "energy signature". Since the human body has a very dynamic energy, the M-Field will shift in both size and symmetry in the presence of other outside energy signatures. How it shifts depends upon the compatibility of the other energies that come within the field influence. The M-field will be attracted to some of the energies, yet be adversely affected by others. Some outside energies make the field expand, while other cause it to contract.

One of the known characteristic of all torus patterns is they tend to be "self-correcting". They each have an inclination toward a specific morphology unique to themselves. Therefore, the energy pattern/energy signature tends to be constant. If distorted for any reason, the torus pattern will attempt to return to its natural state, if given the right resources. For the human body, MFT identifies precisely what those resources are, and provides a measurable outcome as the torus pattern is restored to its optimum fullness and symmetry.

The primary consideration for the MFT practitioner is the size of the *human torus field*, which we call the Morphogenic Field. A large M-Field equates with greater health. The secondary factor that must be considered is the shape of the torus pattern; all sides of the M-Field must be equal when the testing procedure is completed. These two considerations constitute the goals of the MFT Testing Procedure, increase the field size and have it be balanced in the end.

The M-field varies from person to person, just as subjective energy levels do. Some people have very dynamic body energy, while others barely produce enough to get them up in the morning. There are a number of variables that go into the creation of an individual's energy level including age, diet, emotions, stress, exposure to toxins, hydration and physical fitness. Despite these many environmental and behavioral factors, our experience using MFT is constant: the reported level of energy from an individual relates directly to the size and symmetry of their M-Field.

M-Field Signature Matching

Science acknowledges that everything in the universe has its own unique energy signature. Some are consistent, such as inorganic rock, which has the same basic energy signature day after day, month after month, year after year. Meanwhile, organic matter, including plants, animals, and some minerals, have an energy pattern that can be altered radically by seemingly miniscule changes. In the world of quantum physics, it is not possible to totally be in command of the manifestation of an energy signature. However, it is quite easy to alter an energy signature by introducing an artificial substance into a natural environment.

This phenomenon is witnessed regularly in our Wellness Center when performing the MFT signature matching procedure. The addition of the energy of a chemical, toxic heavy metal, or genetically modified food initiates a rapid contraction of the M-Field. Conversely, adding the energy of the exact whole-food nutrients needed by the body causes a rapid expansion of the M-Field. The size of the M-Field is a proxy for the healing ability of the nervous system at that moment in time, and as the M-Field's environment varies, so does the strength and size of the field itself.

Measuring the M-Field

It is possible to objectively measure the size of the M-field as it emanates from the corporeal body. The steps are simple.

For female patients, it begins with a deliberate, methodical introduction of the *energy* of a supplement designed only for the male endocrine (hormone) system to the M-Field. Because the female patient is not a man, her body has no use for the male hormone supplements. The M-Field instantly recognizes this energy "mismatch" and causes a strong test muscle to go weak. If the patient is male, a supplement created exclusively for the female endocrine system is utilized with the same results.

The M-Field will "reject" (the muscle lock will be lost) with mismatched energies and "attract" (the muscle remains locked) with matching energies. When any substance is slowly brought into the Morphogenic Field, a decision is made by the M-Field. If the substance is compatible with the body's energy signature (a *match,* or *attraction*), the test muscle stays strong. If it is incompatible, (a *mismatch,* or *rejection*) the test muscle becomes weak. Although the process is straightforward, it is also remarkably sophisticated, as it reveals information that cannot be discovered any other way.

The measurement is achieved by having the patient estimate the distance from the body where the M-Field responds to the mismatch with a dramatically weakened test muscle. Someone with a very large M-Field (a healthy person) will weaken at a distance of 5 to 7 feet from the actual physical body. A person with a health challenge will see the test muscle weaken from a distance of 0 to 1 feet.

To keep the measurement as objective as possible, the patient declares their observation of the "size", of their M-Field at the start of the procedure. Some people are very good at judging the size of their field; others are "measurement challenged". As a rule, the practitioner operates from whatever measurement is given. The accuracy of the initial measurement is less important than the visual confirmation of a *change* in the size of the field when various new energies are introduced. It is the growth of the M-Field that we are striving for.

After the MFT Testing Procedure is performed, the next phase is to identify the patient's individual nutritional needs. At this point, a skilled practitioner will be able to pinpoint prospective solutions in the form of actual food, whole food supplements, homeopathic remedies or herbal medicines. The proposed supplement-solution is placed into the M-Field, and the muscle response test is performed again. Executed correctly, the M-Field boundary will be measurably larger at the conclusion of the test. A demonstration of this entire process and other facets of the Morphogenic Field Technique can be seen on the MFT website: www.m-field.info.

Genetics versus Epigenetics

From the time of Charles Darwin, scientists believed that all humans were victims of their genetic makeup, that there was one gene for each protein replicated by the body. Since there were approximately 100,000 different proteins, there must therefore be approximately 100,000 genes to direct the replication (Lipton).

The recently completed human genome study found this assumption to be inaccurate. As it turned out, the scientists found less than 25,000 genes when all of the counting was done. This required a shift in thinking and a new direction in research. We now know that a single gene has the ability to influence the replication of up to 2,000 different proteins (Lipton).

As a result of this latest discovery, the new science of *Epigenetics* was born. Epigenetics is the science of *the variables that affect genetic expression*, or, what eventually happens to your genes based upon what you do to them. It turns out we have a lot more power than we thought. But this is a double-edged sword; although we now have some measure of *control* over our genes, we also must *accept responsibility* for our genes.

The factors which affect genetic expression are mostly environmental. How we think, the people we surround ourselves with, and the emotional stresses they introduce are all part of our body environment. The toxins we are exposed to, including chemicals and heavy metals, are also a factor. The content and quality of the food we eat not only affects our daily functioning, it can alter whether or not our genetically predisposed weaknesses become our reality. At some level, most of us already knew this. While it is not an entirely new idea, the Human Genome Project has finally provided the proof. The latest estimate is that approximately 98% of present-day diseases result from environmental factors (Lipton). Of course, there are still ailments that are entirely genetic in nature, such as cystic fibrosis and Huntington's disease. Nonetheless, by creating a healthy climate within our bodies, we can control many of the variables that determine our health as we get older. Our genes are not our fate.

Epigenetic science has also revealed one other important consideration. The way we take care of our genes in this lifetime influences the genetic future of our offspring. Generally speaking, healthy parents create healthy children. This reality also holds true for disease. If we allow our gene pool to degrade, future generations will suffer the consequences.

Over the past two centuries, cultural anthropologists have extensively studied our world's primitive societies. One common factor among these distant cultures was the acute awareness that diet plays an important role in the development of healthy children. The people of these cultures knew this *innately*. There were a number of routines and rituals aimed at ensuring that the young couples, the baby-makers, received the most nutritious food available. The aging females in many societies were responsible for targeting these couples and assisting them in their dietary routines (Price). Survival of their populace depended upon a strong next-generation.

This suggests that the wisdom of Epigenetics was already known by these "simple" peoples. They did not need government-funded research projects to prove it to them. Their innate wisdom over the centuries showed them the right way to perpetuate their species. One might say that these people were the first *Epigeneticists*. Of course, the food that was available to them was real food, the food that today would be labeled as "organic".

Although we have advances in medical science that our ancestors could never dream of, we face a very different type of challenge. Every time a new herbicide is added to the soil, every time a seed is genetically modified, every time there is a chemical manipulation of processing, the energy signature of the food is artificially altered. These changes in the energy signature of the food result in changes to the energy signature of the body. Fortunately, these changes are easy to detect and respond to using the M-Field Energy Signature Matching process.

The Quantum Conversation

To deal with the needs of the body at the cellular level, it involves a *quantum conversation*. The energy signatures of the Morphogenic Field, the MFT Testing Kits, and even the energy of the recommended whole food supplements all represent a "quantum state". Recall that quantum physics is the study of the little pieces of life: the molecules, atoms, subatomic particles and all of the "space" or "field" in-between. The practical application of quantum physics concepts on the three dimensional (3-D) level is difficult to visualize because of the size of atomic particles. Scientists need quantum tools such as the electron microscope in order get a window into this world. Despite their mysterious nature, quantum concepts are fascinating once they are explained in practical terms.

One particularly interesting quantum concept is called "entanglement"; the interactions between seemingly unrelated subatomic energies. A well-known quantum entanglement experiment was performed at the University of Geneva in 1997. A single photon, or light particle, was "split" in two, and each half was sent off in opposite directions down a fiber-optic line for a distance of 7 miles. At the end of this line, the split photon had the option of turning right or left. Although these disconnected halves were now 14 miles apart, when the option to turn left or right occurred, each particle always chose the same direction as its counterpart. (Braden)

In the theory of quantum entanglement, there remains a "connectedness" even when the parts are separated by great distance. This type of entanglement phenomenon occurs frequently in nature; disconnected, yet still connected. Even though there is no obvious "hardwired" connection, each cell of your body is entangled with every other cell, and they are in communication at all times. With the Morphogenic Field Technique, we have the opportunity to be a part of that communication, of that *quantum conversation*, to identify which foods truly support the needs of our bodies.

For the practical application of MFT, one must be able to acknowledge the quantum field that manifests from the body. Perhaps a quantum physicist could provide a detailed explanation of its exact nature, but most MFT practitioners simply develop a feel for it. As with gravity, you can see it work but you can't see IT. Similar to magnetism, you can see the results of it, but you cannot see IT. After working with the Morphogenic Field for many years, I feel it and I know it exists in the same way I know gravity and magnetism exist. More compelling than my story though, are the stories of the patients who have experienced the incredible healing power of the Morphogenic Field Technique firsthand.

Chantéa's Story

> When I came into Dr. Springob's office in September 2011, I had crippling, 24/7 fetal-positioned stomach pain, headaches, dizziness, severe malnutrition, weight loss, weakness and insomnia; all of which I had suffered from for over two years, steadily becoming worse. I was in such an extreme amount

of pain that I couldn't even clap my hands because it jarred my body too much.

Hospital after hospital, clinic after clinic, I had been seen by medical professionals in three different states and no one could find anything wrong with me. Since doctors could not figure out the problem, again and again they would prescribe me pain medication and turn me away, which was absolutely devastating to me because I knew that it was only a remedy to mask the pain. Because I recognized the damage that these drugs cause for organs and the addictions that could ensue, I refused to take the narcotics and opted for a more natural treatment, but even then I would often have to take doses every two to three hours just to walk normally or even stand up straight. Even though I never spoke the words, I knew I was literally dying.

In what I believe to be divine orchestration, I had actually had a background with Dr. Frank Springob as I had gone to high school in Port Angeles, WA; being the multi-sport athlete that I was, I had been seen by him for chiropractic therapy. At one point in November of 2010 I came to visit Port Angeles for my brother's wedding and my mom scheduled me for a visit to see Dr. Frank. In that one appointment he had found the "energy" of a microbe in my small intestines and gave me an antidote for it, but since I had lived in California at the time I wasn't able to have any kind of monitoring or follow up. After using the remedy for the microbe energy I began to get increasingly better, but within two months I hit a plateau and then spiraled back down again. It wasn't until almost a year later that I made the decision to move back to Port Angeles for as long as it would take for me to be thoroughly treated and cured.

The first visit back we discovered the source of my problem: I was being "eaten alive". Dr. Frank's testing procedure indicated the energy of parasitic worms in my system. By describing to him all of my specific symptoms and using his method of reading the messages my body was emitting, he was able to discern that not only were the "critters" in my small intestine, but they were in my heart and brain as well. It was an absolute miracle I was even alive! He recommended different specifically formulated nutrient supplements that would kill the parasites and began to rebuild me at the cellular level back to health.

Within five months of addressing the root of my illness and malnutrition, layer after layer, I was able to walk, run, jump and truly smile again. I am 100% pain free, a feeling that during those two years I had sincerely forgotten. I'm finally back to being my normal, energetic and agile self. I can't tell you how many visits it took for me to stop crying out of sheer gratefulness while he was working with me because I was finally seeing hope again and experiencing actual healing. I am just so thankful, because through this man, The Lord gave my life back to me.

Chapter 4

The Food Story

Where We Have Been and What We Ate Along the Way

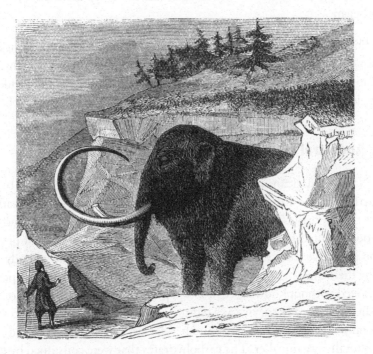

Question: How do you eat an elephant?
Answer: One bite at a time, of course!

My hometown of Port Angeles is located approximately 15 miles from a famous archeological dig, the Manis Mastadon Site, unearthed in 1977. According to the scientific journal "Science", this location is the oldest human settlement the Western Hemisphere found to date. There, tools and artifacts have been dated back to 13,800 years ago, older than the Clovis Site in New Mexico by 1000 years. The dig at the Manis Mastodon site uncovered the remains of bison, caribou, and elk, but the nearly 14,000 year old mastodon remains the big attraction at the visitor's center.

I recall reading about the discovery in the local newspaper when it was first publicized, trying to imagine the early humans' relationship to this beast. It was found with a spear point embedded in its side, confirming for archaeologists that humans were indeed hunting in this area at that time. I was reminded of the old joke about how to eat an elephant, which I have referred to many times in my life when faced with a large, daunting project. Breaking things down into smaller pieces makes them manageable, and it is the approach I used in my research on the story of where our local food began.

A fitting analogy, since so close to my home there is an actual historical settlement where people literally "ate the elephant" for survival. Right here in Happy Valley, just south of Sequim, Washington, lays ample evidence of the known origins of the traditional diet in the Western Hemisphere.

The Ancestral Diet and the Modern Diet

The Native American indigenous people survived many millennia before the arrival of the European settlers to "the New World." Tribal nations across the country consumed the food that was available to them, and it is well documented that there was an abundance of animal fat and protein in the primitive diet. Less obvious, perhaps, is the fact that nobody was getting their cholesterol checked on a regular basis. 14,000 years ago, people functioned without knowing their blood pressure or their resting heart rate. Yet, they managed to survive as a culture for thousands of years. Of course, the food was devoid of pesticides and herbicides; what today we would refer to as a totally organic diet. The carbohydrates that were consumed by early humans were in their complex form, since refined carbohydrates would not exist for another 13,400 years. Somewhere in that span of time, our diet and our way of thinking about food changed radically.

We do a different sort of hunting now. In the 21st Century, conscientious shoppers spend a lot of time reading the labels on the food for sale at the grocery store. For those who are interested in health, the goal of the hunt is to find a nutrient-rich, high quality organic food supply. Today, this type of food can seem more elusive than a mastodon. As consumers we must decipher, from reading labels on packages, whether or not the contents are something we really want to put into our mouths.

The Native American ancestors who occupied the Happy Valley village 14 millennia ago had no such worries. Whatever maladies they may have suffered as a culture, cancer was probably not one of them. Now we live in a world where it comes as no surprise to learn that something we have been eating, breathing or cleaning with is a known or possible carcinogen. While regulatory agencies try to limit the exposure of the known carcinogens that we consume, these limits often come only after decades of exposure to the offending substance.

Big agribusiness and the chemical industry introduce thousands of new artificial chemicals into food supply and the greater environment every year. Much of this is done without sufficient testing to evaluate the risks of exposing the population to potential threats. Regulatory agencies have explained that extensive safety studies are not practical; it would be too expensive and it would slow the progress of new products to the market. While you and I may believe that delaying the marketing of new chemicals is a great idea, it is likely that DuPont and Dow Chemical do not. Rather than proving the safety of a new product prior to introduction to the public, the product must be proven to be unsafe before it is "pulled" from the market. In the meantime, we are all exposed to it. This is not the recipe for another 14,000 years of survival.

More Ancestral Food

Fourteen millennia ago, nature provided enough of what was needed that Native American Tribal Nations such as the Makah, the S'Klallam, the Quinault, the Hoh and the Quileute still inhabit the Olympic Peninsula to this day. In fact, just 70 miles in the other direction from Port Angeles, there is another famous archeological site, the Ozette Site. Located at Cape Alava, the westernmost point in the continental United States, the Ozette Site features a long-buried Native American longhouse that was discovered in the early 1970s. It is postulated that this building was engulfed by a landslide in approximately the mid 1700's. Many of the perfectly preserved

27

artifacts removed from the site are on display in a museum on the reservation of the Makah Nation in Neah Bay, Washington.

The archaeological excavation of the site took over a decade, during which a great deal was learned about the traditional ways of the Makah ancestors. The unearthing of this early history spawned a resurgence of appreciation for the traditional ways among the Makah people over the past few decades. Despite the lengthy depreciation of the accumulated dietary and cultural wisdom of this ancient society that occurred following the arrival of the European settlers, there is an obvious pride in their heritage. Many traditional dances and other cultural events are held on a regular basis and the native language is again being taught in their schools.

The discovery of the buried longhouse at the Ozette site provided more information about the food supply of the indigenous people of the Olympic Peninsula 13,500 years after that mastodon was killed in Happy Valley. For the purposes of traditional food research, these two sites serve as "bookends" to compare the longstanding dietary commonalities. Looking at the diet of both settlements, we can project similarities in the diet of all of the Native Americans that lived on the Olympic Peninsula for those 13,500 years.

While animal protein sources were the primary sustenance for both civilizations, the greatest change came from the addition of foods from the ocean. The Ozette site provided ample evidence that salmon, halibut, clams, crab, whale, seal, kelp and other food harvested from the sea were prominent dietary resources. As one Makah Tribal elder, Gary Ray, told me during a conversation at our Wellness Center recently, "They ate from the forest early in the day and ate from the ocean late in the day".

The Great Diet Change

Many dietary changes have come about since the white man entered the scene on the northwest coast approximately 150 years ago. At that time, a dramatic alteration in the traditional diet was thrust upon the native people. Although a few of the Makah Elders can still recall some of the traditional eating practices, much of what is known about the ancestral diet was learned at the archeological site at Cape Alava. The changes in dietary habits also affected the settlers, as it was coincidentally about

150 years ago when food processing changed across America as a whole, becoming gradually more industrial and less nutritious.

Comparing traditional diets of primitive societies with the diet of modern America is not a new idea. This concept was explored extensively by Dr. Weston Price in the 1930's. In the early decades of the 20th century, Dr. Price was a practicing dentist who was disturbed by a trend he saw in his patients. Over three decades, the integrity of the dental structure in the general public seemed to be deteriorating. He was particularly disturbed with the increase in dental caries (cavities) and weakening of the jaw structure.

Dr. Price theorized that the origin of these problems coincided with the increase in consumption of commercial food. As the population in the early 20th Century ate more refined and processed foods, Dr. Price believed that these "foods of commerce" did not provide the nutrients required for a strong healthy body. He theorized that food degradation was the reason for the increasing dental deterioration. He was interested in finding the secret of which type of diet would consistently provide true health.

For 10 years, Dr. Price and his wife traveled around the world looking for populations of people from societies that remained untouched by the new commercial world. In his quest to learn and document the diets of the healthiest people throughout the world, the Price's visited hundreds of settlements in 14 different countries. This same research project would be almost impossible to repeat today, given the reach of the processed food industry.

During this endeavor, Dr. Price visited some remote areas, including the southwest coast of Vancouver Island. Although the Olympic Peninsula, the subject of this discussion, was not one of his destinations, it is well documented that the aboriginal people of Vancouver Island are related to the tribes of the North Olympic Peninsula. They shared many traditions, native plants, and food sources.

Dr. Price's Findings

Dr. Price's 10 year research project led to the creation of an inventory of dietary factors present in every traditional food supply. This list contains immutable rules that must be obeyed in every society for long-term health and propagation of the species, and has been adapted to address the dietary options of the present day. This list comes directly from the Weston A. Price Foundation:

The 11 Characteristics of Traditional Diets

1. The diets of healthy, non-industrialized peoples contain no refined or denatured foods or ingredients, such as refined sugar or high fructose corn syrup; white flour; canned foods; pasteurized, homogenized, skim or low-fat milk; refined or hydrogenated vegetable oils; protein powders; artificial vitamins; or toxic additives and colorings.

2. All traditional cultures consume some sort of animal food, such as fish and shellfish; land and water fowl; land and sea mammals; eggs; milk and milk products; reptiles; and insects. The whole animal is consumed—muscle meat, organs, bones and fat, with the organ meats and fats preferred.

3. The diets of healthy, non-industrialized peoples contain at least four times the minerals and water soluble vitamins, and 10 times the fat soluble vitamins found in animal fats as the average American diet.

4. All traditional cultures cooked some of their food but all consumed a portion of their animal foods raw.

5. Primitive and traditional diets have a high content of food enzymes and beneficial bacteria from lacto-fermented vegetables, fruits, beverages, dairy products, meats and condiments.

6. Seeds, grains and nuts are soaked, sprouted, fermented or naturally leavened to neutralize naturally occurring anti-nutrients such as enzyme inhibitors, tannins and phytic acid.

7. Total fat content of traditional diets varies from 30% to 80% of calories but only about 4% of calories come from polyunsaturated oils naturally occurring in grains, legumes, nuts, fish, animal fats and vegetables. The balance of fat calories is in the form of saturated and mono-unsaturated fatty acids.

8. Traditional diets contain nearly equal amounts of omega-6 and omega-3 essential fatty acids.

9. All traditional diets contain some salt.

10. All traditional cultures make use of animal bones, especially in the form of gelatin-rich bone broths.

11. Traditional cultures make provisions for the health of future generations by providing special nutrient-rich animal foods for parents-to-be, pregnant women and growing children; by proper spacing of children; and by teaching the principles of right diet to the young.

Finding These Foods

Weston Price's research has given the world a great gift by identifying a cross-cultural baseline for a nutritious, sustainable diet that has allowed for the survival of the species for thousands of years. He published these findings in 1939 in his landmark book, "Nutrition and Physical Degeneration." Currently in print through the Price-Pottenger Nutrition Foundation, this book is a must read for anyone looking for answers about the nutritional needs of the human body.

Dr. Price's 11 item inventory can be used to assess any diet for nutritional completeness. Along with a comprehensive literature review, interviews with tribal elders, and investigation of local ethno-botanical resources, the above list served as a model by which to evaluate the known traditional diet of the indigenous people of the Olympic Peninsula. Research revealed that their eating habits were consistent with Dr. Price's findings in every respect.

The existence of fermented foods was verified by Gary Ray, the Makah Tribal elder, who explained how salmon eggs were put into baskets and buried underground for the winter to ferment. He stated, "There was a traditional ceremony held annually where the fermented eggs (a sort of caviar) would be consumed with the fresh new green sprouts in the spring". Gay Hunter, Curator of the Cultural Resources Department of Olympic National Park, provided invaluable books describing traditional fermented foods consumed by local tribes including the Makah, the S'Klallam, and the Quinault. Fermented sources included wine from cranberries, berries stored in baskets and consumed after turning brown from fermentation, and crab apples cooked in water and then stored for later use in a fermented state (Gunther, Moerman,Wray). Other Makah elders related oral traditions that included the fermentation of both whale blubber and seal oil.

In the typical modern American diet, beneficial bacteria may come to us in the form of foods such as live-culture yogurt, sauerkraut, pickles, or sourdough bread, provided they are made in the traditional, lacto-fermented method. Fermented foods provide a multitude of digestive advantages, a fact that even the American Dietetic Association acknowledges. However, most of the options available on supermarket shelves are imposters. To find authentic, lacto-fermented foods, consumers must be savvy enough to discern the difference or creative enough to make their own.

Another feature of Dr. Price's research that often comes as a surprise to mainstream American consumers is the inclusion of raw or "undercooked" protein as an important nutritional source. The current predominant belief is that all "bacteria" needs to be killed by the cooking process for fear that consuming undercooked meat could have dire consequences.

This fear was magnified by a well-publicized case of E. coli infection originating from a Seattle area fast food restaurant in 1993. Undercooked hamburger was implicated as the cause of the outbreak, and thoroughly cooking it was stressed as the solution in the news reports at that time. The origin of that particular E. coli outbreak was discovered, yet the core problems with the fast food supply infrastructure remain largely unaddressed.

The rarely talked about problem is that fast food restaurants utilize factory-farmed beef as their source of hamburger. In the commercial world of cattle rearing, cows are kept in a small enclosure called a "feedlot", which is an unnatural environment for them. Cows are traditionally pastured animals that eat grass, not grain. Grain-fed cattle raised on feed lots are prone to bacterial infections, which are controlled by the periodic application of antibiotic therapy. The antibiotics also make their way into the meat. The resulting commercial meat has an energy signature quite different from that of beef that has been naturally raised, grass fed, and pastured without the use of antibiotics. While Dr. Price's study tells us that there is nutritional benefit to consuming undercooked meat, eating animals raised in a perverse factory-farmed environment can indeed be harmful to your health. Overcooking *is* a prudent way to insure that the microbes that tend to be present in commercial meat are eradicated.

However, it important to note that excessive over-cooking of meat can have negative health consequences over the long-term. Over-cooking can destroy certain "heat-labile" amino acids which are necessary for building the protein in our bodies. Protein is made-up of chains of amino acids, all of which must all be available during the *protein creation* process in the body. If the required amino acids are unavailable due to over-cooking, physical degeneration can result.

Dr. Price's observations of the necessity of some dietary source of raw or under-cooked meat have since been confirmed in other research. The most well-known studies on this subject were performed in the 1940's by Dr. Francis Pottenger, who demonstrated extreme physical degeneration in cats fed diets deficient in heat-labile amino acids. Although there were other factors tested, Pottenger's study found that over-cooked protein accelerated the process of physical degeneration to the point where, within three generations, the cats could no longer reproduce. Consequently, the testing came to an end.

Based upon his findings with cats, Dr. Pottenger predicted similar reproductive issues may arise in the human population within a few generations. According to noted fertility specialist Dr. Iva Keene, infertility is now "an alarming epidemic affecting more couples than ever. One out of six couples today experience difficulty falling pregnant. What was once seen as a woman's problem is now known to affect men equally."(Mercola)

The White Man's Store

In his book, Dr. Price tells the story of the search for scurvy among the indigenous people in Canada. Through an interpreter he asked a tribal member whether or not it was possible for the Indian to get scurvy. The response was that scurvy was a white man's disease, but yes, it was possible. The Native Canadian added that the Indian knows how to prevent scurvy and the white man does not. At first he would not share the secret with Dr. Price. When asked repeatedly why he would not share the secret, the Indian replied that the white man knew too much to ask the Indian anything.

Dr. Price continued to press the issue and finally got the Indian to agree that he would tell if the Chief said it was alright. He went to see the chief and upon returning, he told Dr. Price that the chief had agreed since Dr. Price was a friend to the Indians, because he had told them not to eat the food from the white man's store.

The Indian then described how when a moose is killed, they open it up and find the gland above the kidney, which we call the adrenal gland. He said this gland would be cut up into little pieces and distributed to families based upon the number of family members, who each got one piece. This is how the Indian prevents scurvy, Dr. Price was told. In modern times, we now know that the adrenal gland has the richest store of vitamin C complex in the body. It is an established fact that vitamin C complex prevents scurvy. Although no scientist had ever disclosed this fact to these people, they already had the innate knowledge that this was so.

The "Value" of the Traditional Diet

In analyzing the diet of the indigenous people, the ones he called the "Northern Indians", Dr. Price formed some of his conclusions about the nutrition levels available to that population versus that of a modernized diet of the 1930's. It was noted that the Northern Indians diet contained 5.8 times the calcium, 5.8 times the phosphorus, 2.7 times the iron, 4.3 times the magnesium, 1.5 times the copper and 8.8 times the iodine of the modernized diet. Because he was a dentist, the focus on dental health is evident in his findings. In these indigenous people, the percentage of teeth with dental caries was less than one-fifth of 1%.

This is striking when compared to the modernized diet of the 1930's, where 21.5% of the teeth had cavities. This translates to an epidemic of cavities over 80 times greater in the modern "civilized" areas. Although these primitive people did not have access to the modern dental hygiene habits that we take for granted such as fluoride, brushing, flossing, rinsing and regular check-ups, they naturally had incredibly strong teeth because of a diet that did not promote tooth decay.

If the traditional diet of primitive people could create this kind of result in dental health, it raises the question: What about the other systems of the body? The high quality nutrition of the indigenous people allowed for equally high quality dental health. We know that all systems of the body require high quality nutrition, because the nutrients in food are the building blocks of the body. Today, almost 80 years after Dr. Price completed his research, it is well documented that the nutritional value of our current food supply is less than half of what it was back then. Commercial soil is so depleted of minerals that it now takes 65 cups of spinach to provide the level of iron that one cup provided in 1945. An orange that contained 50 mg. of vitamin C complex in 1950 now contains 5 mg. (Frost) Modern agricultural practices have done nothing to reverse this trend, so based on this pattern, we can extrapolate that overall we consume approximately 10% of the nutrients ingested 150 years ago. Today, most of us have been shopping at the "white man's store".

Many of the Makah and S'Klallam tribal members are attempting to reproduce their traditional diet to the best of their ability. I've treated some of these people for almost four decades. The MFT Procedure encourages biochemical individuality, which means paying attention to the ancestral diet. Although this way of thinking has improved the health of all of my patients, the lure of refined commercial products is everywhere, and no one is immune to the intense marketing gimmicks.

I have always believed in the principles of free will and choice. Everybody has the opportunity to improve themselves or waste away as they choose, but those choices should be based upon knowledge of what is healthy or unhealthy. In the matter of modern junk food, the manipulative nature of the marketing makes it difficult for people to make good choices, and government endorsement of unsound farming practices leaves us all confused to say the least.

The Modern Food Challenge

There are many examples of modern food processing and industrial agricultural practices which have altered our genetics, our teeth, and every aspect of our health. Sadly, this decline has been happening on a routine basis in the United States for over a century. In 1906, President Theodore Roosevelt instituted the Pure Food and Drug Act. This resolution was based largely upon the scientific work of Dr. Harvey W. Wiley, chief of the USDA's Bureau of Chemistry. Although enacted to protect the American consumer, the law was soon radically changed by commercial interests with great political influence.

In spite of Supreme Court rulings that upheld the Food and Drug Law, the ruling was effectively ignored by USDA Secretary James Wilson. By 1931, Dr. Wiley's Bureau of Chemistry had evolved into the Food and Drug Administration, headed by Dr. Elmer M. Nelson. Dr. Nelson became notorious for pushing court decisions that blocked health food manufacturers from differentiating the quality of real food from that of processed or synthetic food to the public. (Frost)

The intention of President Roosevelt was to insure that future generations would not have to be concerned with the safety and quality of their food supply. Unfortunately, President Woodrow Wilson's cabinet operated to protect the commercial food and drug industries at the expense of the people. Since that time, political appointments to these regulatory organizations have often been derived from political contributions, alliances, and cronyism.

A standout example of this is found in the Obama administration. Despite campaign promises made by then-Senator Obama to push for legislation to require the labeling of genetically modified foods, no such legislation has been introduced. In fact, in an act that seemed to contradict the campaign promise, Obama instead appointed Michael Taylor as "Food Czar" at the FDA. Mr. Taylor has a rich history with Monsanto, the giant chemical corporation that created many of the genetically modified seeds in current use. It was Michael Taylor who, in 1992, authored the FDA policy on genetically modified foods. The Statement of Policy reads:

> **"The agency is not aware of any information showing that food derived by these new methods differs from other foods in any meaningful or uniform way."**

This policy has remained intact for the past 20 years despite strong vocal opposition from the FDA's own scientists, who expressed dismay that this obvious political statement was not backed by any valid science. Many of them were fired or censured for openly questioning a policy that has been proven to be erroneous in multiple studies done by a variety of entities, including Monsanto (Smith).

Mr. Taylor was an attorney at Monsanto prior to writing the FDA policy on GMO's in 1992. Afterward, he returned to Monsanto in the role of vice president. Currently, he is back at the FDA serving as the man in charge of our food safety. Lack of integrity in government agencies is nothing new, but this "corporate-to-agency revolving door" creates incestuous relationships that breed perverse policies. It has become increasingly clear that the people of the United States cannot depend upon the government regulatory agencies that were created to protect our health and our environment.

There is a palpable shift taking place in this country. An increasing level of discontent within the ranks of average Americans can be seen in the "Occupy" demonstrations. People are recognizing that the decisions made behind closed doors benefit only a very small percentage of the populous, and they are confronting the political status quo. The Occupy movement was organized in response to corruption in the American financial system, and this same awareness is brewing among the citizens concerned with the state of our food supply.

MFT empowers an ordinary person to take back their health in a way that cannot be controlled or manipulated for the benefit of any corporation or stockholder. MFT is truly Natural Health Care of the people, by the people, and for the people. The premise is simple: ask the body what it needs, and then give it what it asks for!

Chapter 5

Frank's Story

"The important thing is not to stop questioning. Curiosity has its own reason for existing."

~Albert Einstein

My First Visit to the Chiropractor

My perspective on health care began at the age of 10. There were many days when I would come home from school with excruciating headaches. I still recall arriving at the house, going to my bedroom, closing the window curtains and crying because my head hurt so badly. My mother, who was pregnant with my youngest brother, had been seeing a chiropractor for back and neck pain related to the pregnancy. Dr. Jennings worked out of a small office in Mountlake Terrace, Washington. At that time, he was approximately 85 years old, and had been in practice for over 60 years.

A graduate of Palmer School of Chiropractic, Dr. Jennings told my mother that there were six people in his graduating class. The training at that time was approximately six months long, and his lone instructor was Dr. D.D. Palmer, the founder of the chiropractic profession. My mother asked Dr. Jennings about the headaches that I was having. Could chiropractic do anything to help with my excruciating pain? Dr. Jennings encouraged her to bring me into his office. She'd gotten so much relief from her back pain that she agreed to bring me back later that week.

Now, 50 years later, I still recall the small dark office. As you came through the front door, the most striking thing was a wall mounting with a sign that said "Take a Number". Dr. Jennings did not have a receptionist and there was no evidence of a telephone. The appointment system was very simple: you came in, you took a number--- first come, first served.

I will always remember my first impression of Dr. Jenning's office. The lighting was dim, there was a lack of decoration, and an old radiator stood out in the corner. I remember Dr. Jennings warming his hands over that radiator prior to placing them on my spine as I lay on a simple table. However, the object that grabbed the attention of my 10 year old mind above all else was the skeleton in the corner.

As I lay down on the table, the old chiropractor began probing up and down my spine with a touch so gentle that I wondered what he could possibly be feeling. My father was there and explained about my headaches during a brief history. As Dr. Jennings was palpating my spine, he started reciting other symptoms I was probably having based on what he was feeling. He had not been told of the symptoms because I had not complained about them; he just seemed to know exactly what I was feeling.

I could not understand at the time how could he possibly know about the stomach problems I was having. The old chiropractor asked me if I got lightheaded if I stood up too fast. "How could he tell that by just touching me?" I wondered. He seemed to know where all of my sore spots were. Although I did not fully understand what was going on, when it was over I felt as if a great pressure had been relieved. Although I could not have been sure at that moment, from that time on the headaches became much less of a problem in my life. In my mind, the obvious conclusion was that chiropractors existed to get rid of headaches.

Periodically, I returned for follow-up visits. Approximately six months later, Dr. Jennings was no longer showing up in his office. Within another month, I heard that he had passed away. With my headaches now gone, it would be several years before I again visited a chiropractor.

The Career Path

I began my professional career in a quandary. During my senior year in high school, my friend Lance and I spent an afternoon in his rec room looking through the class catalog from the University of Washington. Since we both had a high school background in the sciences, we mutually felt that looking at various science majors was a good place to start when thinking about the future.

The year was 1970. Our choices were limited by the fact that neither one of us was particularly interested in being drafted by the U.S. Army. At that time, one thing was perfectly clear to us: if we were not enrolled in college, within a matter of months we would get a letter of "greetings" from Uncle Sam. Those were the days of the Vietnam War. Many of our high school classmates would soon be receiving their draft notice. Lance and I had no intention of having this happen to us; therefore, our only recourse was to attend college.

Given the situation, the logical thing to do was to throw darts. We placed the names of all the seemingly acceptable majors offered at the University of Washington on Lance's dartboard. We made an agreement that where that dart landed would dictate our futures. It landed on "Pharmacy". True to our agreement, we both applied for and were accepted at the University Washington School of Pharmacy. Six years later, Lance graduated with a pharmacy degree, whereas I lasted about one month.

That was the month that changed my life.

As I sat in the introductory pharmacy classes, it became apparent to me that I had no future within this profession. My first clue came during one of the lectures in the first days of the first quarter. The professor mentioned a few of the types of drugs available for headache pain. I made a casual remark that I visited the chiropractor whenever I had a headache. I was not prepared for what was about to follow.

The professor took it upon himself to expend a great deal of time and energy to let me know, in no uncertain terms, that chiropractors were unscientific quacks. Although it was obvious to me that this man knew very little about chiropractic, he had absolutely no qualms about voicing an opinion on the subject.

I was stunned by his statements. I knew I had gotten a great deal of relief from my headaches, yet I was now being told that what I believed could not possibly be true. It was at this point that I began to question the integrity of the profession that I was about to enter. I had always been told by my parents that one should not express an opinion on a subject of which one has no knowledge. I considered the professor's behavior extremely unprofessional.

This event, in and of itself, was not sufficient to get me to reject my career path since it was only the ranting of one individual. But it did alert me to the possibility that the "pharmaceutical truth" was not necessarily my truth.

The Parting Truth

Concurrently, I sat through several lectures discussing the different types of pharmacy-related careers. I was particularly impacted by a guest lecture from the representative of a major pharmaceutical company who had come to deliver the career perspective of a pharmaceutical salesman. He stated that he preferred to think of himself as an educator to the medical profession.

Essentially, the drug "rep" talked about visiting the offices of medical doctors and providing them with free drug samples, literature and *incentives* to write prescriptions for whatever patented drug he was showcasing on that particular visit. One of the incentives included conference vacations to exotic places such as Hawaii or the Caribbean, should the M.D. meet certain prescription quotas. Doctors who wrote more than 50 prescriptions over a certain time could qualify for an all-expense-paid educational trip.

During this same lecture, the pharmaceutical company representative alluded to *sales goals* regarding how many doses of the medication they could aim to sell annually at the national level. The numbers of doses ran into the millions per day. This may not be surprising to people who are familiar with the sales tactics of the pharmaceutical industry. However, at that time I was a young, idealistic, college student and I was appalled that it just seemed to be an industry-wide numbers game.

In applying for pharmacy school, I believed I was going into a profession that was interested in improving the health of the American public. Even though this experience occurred more than 40 years ago, the memory of my emotional reaction to that lecture is still ever-present my brain. The primary motivation was to see how many pills they could sell and at what price. This drug rep did not seem to be interested in the impact on the users of the product he was selling. Never once did he speak of healing, health, or improved quality of life.

I had spent much of the previous month listening to lectures about side effects and adverse reactions to some medications. Additionally, I had been exposed early on to the pharmaceutical/medical profession's ignorance and prejudice toward the concepts of natural healing. The primary question in my mind on that day was the integrity of the entire medical industry. I wanted to believe that health care should be about health.

 I recalled reading the novel, *Catch 22,* by Joseph Heller. In that book, the main character, an American World War II bombardier, had to report to the squadron physician. In the dialog, the doctor kept referring to his profession as the "medical business". Up until that time, I'd considered the healing professions to be a much higher calling than just another "business".

Dr. Kildare, the television physician of my youth, had seemed like such a great guy. These few weeks of experience in Pharmacy School now led me to question lifelong beliefs. I left the University of Washington campus that day, never to return. Without even bothering to withdraw from school, I just walked away.

One month later, my mother received a call from the university. Someone had realized that I was no longer there and they were wondering what had happened to me. The caller explained to my mother that I was not attending class. My mother explained to the caller that she was aware and that I would not be returning. The university employee then informed my mother that I had to return to campus to "officially" withdraw from school. When I returned the call to the university, it initiated a very odd conversation, to say the least.

I was told by the person of the other end of the line that I must drive the 3 hours to Seattle from my home in Port Angeles and officially withdraw. I stated that I had no intention of returning to the campus, adding that if withdrawing was required, they should take it upon themselves to withdraw me. The lady on the other end of the phone politely, though desperately, explained to me that if I did not return to Seattle and officially withdrawn in person, I would never again be allowed to enroll at the University of Washington.

The conversation ended when I repeated that I would not be making the trip to Seattle. To this day, I still do not know my official status at UW.

A New Path

The next step in my career was to get the prerequisites required to attend Chiropractic College. Even though I was unsure if I had a future in this healing profession, the shock of the pharmaceutical lecture stuck with me. Chiropractic was the antithesis of Pharmacy. There were no drugs involved in chiropractic. I had decided that natural health care would be my next path, for better or for worse.

I will admit that in the beginning I doubted my new career choice. I moved to Iowa in the autumn of 1972 to enroll in Palmer College of Chiropractic, the same school that Dr. Jennings had attended. In the first quarter, Chiropractic Philosophy was the first class of the day. Dr. Galen Price was the professor. Although I never knew his age, I would guess that he was in his late 70's or early 80's at that time. He was an old friend of the Palmer Family and he still had an active practice. His love of the chiropractic profession was evident.

The purpose of the Chiropractic Philosophy class was to orient students from various backgrounds to the uniqueness of chiropractic thought. We began by learning that healing came from "the top down and the inside out". We also learned that "the Power that made the body, heals the body". We heard about the concept of *Universal Intelligence* and we studied another concept, *Innate Intelligence*. Dr. Galen Price's implication was that Universal Intelligence meant God (or your interpretation of God), while Innate Intelligence was the more individualized version; the "God Within".

At first, I saw this simplistic philosophy as a professional weakness. Now, as the years have gone by, I have come to see this as an elegant truth and an incredible professional strength. The chiropractic profession can be proud of its unfaltering ability to see the human body in terms of an organism that will heal itself unless something is *stopping that from happening*.

In those years, I considered myself a man of science. Even though I had personal experience with the healing power of the chiropractic adjustment, I felt that Dr. Price's explanations seemed inadequate to justify the results I had experienced. Forty years ago I believed that the chiropractic profession had a responsibility to research the results achieved through a chiropractic adjustment and explain it in more scientific terms.

Now, after 36 years of chiropractic practice, and witnessing many miracles I cannot explain, my view has softened. I still consider science to be incredibly important, but we cannot argue with the wisdom of the body. We do not have to understand something in order for it to be true; sometimes it just *is*. It appears the scientific community is beginning to come to this same conclusion, as even respected journals use the term "intelligent design" to define much of the phenomenon they have yet to be able to fully explain.

Exposure to Nutrition

Dr. D.D. Palmer published a book in 1914: *The Chiropractic Adjustor*. In his book he introduced many of his beliefs regarding healing in the human body, which formed the foundation of the chiropractic profession. Dr. Palmer used the terminology of that era to explain various "blockages" to healing, including the words "traumatism" to describe mechanical issues with the body, "poisons" to describe chemical imbalances, and "autosuggestion" to describe emotional stress.

With these words, Dr. Palmer explained to his colleagues that health was comparable to a *triangle*. All three of these areas (mechanics, biochemistry and emotions) needed to be in balance for total health. This later came to be described as the chiropractic "triangle of health". Although this description is now almost 100 years old, it remains a valuable foundational model for interpreting health and wellness.

Despite my initial skepticism of the intuitive nature of chiropractic healing, it eventually became obvious to me the triangle of health provided a framework to understand my patients who were slow to heal. The question became, which side of the triangle was out-of-balance?

The "poison" side of the triangle, the body chemistry, also came to represent the issues of nutritional deficiency. The food has changed a great deal since the advent of the triangle in 1914. This modern refined and processed food contains many humanly-altered factors that Dr. Palmer never had to deal with, including additives and preservatives, trans-fats, and an overabundance of refined sugar. Even forty years ago, when I was studying in Chiropractic College, we were not yet faced with the additional challenges of high fructose corn syrup and genetically modified seeds.

The beginning of my exposure to solutions for nutritional deficiencies came from my chiropractic school roommate, Meed West. Also from the state of Washington, Meed had been taking classes from fellow students studying the new muscle testing science of Applied Kinesiology (AK). Developed by Dr. George Goodheart, a chiropractor from Michigan, this new discipline linked the different skeletal muscles and their nerve supply to corresponding organs (Walther). These classes were not taught on the Palmer campus, since they were not part of the core curriculum, but I learned enough about AK to understand the application and to treat certain specific nutritional issues.

In fact, Meed and I used Dr. Goodheart's spinal analysis testing before I delivered my very first chiropractic adjustment in 1973. The patient was one of Meed's old high school buddies, Earl, who was living in Chicago. We were visiting the city for the Memorial Day weekend and staying at Earl's apartment. Earl complained that his neck was sore, and I was more than eager to test out my newfound chiropractic adjusting skills while Meed assisted me with the AK analysis. In the end, Dr. Goodheart's analysis proved invaluable for guiding my intervention with Earl, who said he felt much better after the treatment. AK got me off to a good start as a chiropractor.

The "Business" Realization

I opened my chiropractic practice in 1976 in Port Angeles. Slowly, the practice grew, but I spent much of my first few years in survival mode. There were always more bills than there was money. It took approximately seven years before the situation reversed. It was during that time that I realized that chiropractic, too, was a business. In order to help patients heal, I had to first keep the doors open.

On one occasion a new patient appeared with a rather serious spinal condition. After a history and examination, I explained the serious nature of this problem to the patient. I stressed the intense level of care required to resolve his pain and stabilize his spine. Fortunately, the patient had very good insurance. Unfortunately, I had a fleeting thought that this person's problem would help me pay some of my high office overhead.

The very fact that I had considered this to be an advantageous situation left me feeling guilty that I would profit from another person's suffering. I remember having a talk with my wife Linda about my "relationship with my patients" versus "my relationship with my fees". We came to the agreement that I would be kept in the dark when it came to patient accounts. In this way, I could spend my time thinking only about the well-being of the patients and money would not be a consideration in their care.

There was something about that event that forced me to recall my reaction to the presentation by the pharmaceutical company representative at the University of Washington all those years before. If health care was just another business, then was I just another businessman.

My wife Linda, also my office manager all these years, has always held to this agreement. She may be aware that any given patient has an outstanding balance owing, but I am not. If I run into somebody on the street, I can always be happy to see them and sincerely ask them how they are doing. I do not know if I *would*, but I *might* treat them differently if I knew they owed me money. Fortunately for me, Linda has been there for me all these years to shoulder that responsibility. It has helped me tremendously to have her there to confront the issue of patient finances so that I could focus on the healing.

Finding My Way Back

By the mid 1980's, we were no longer in survival mode. The practice had grown to the point where we were paying our bills comfortably and had enough left over for an occasional vacation. It was at this point that I decided to further explore the nutrition component in my practice. The state of Washington had very strict laws in those days for chiropractors. Basically, the chiropractic practice law outlined all the things **we could not do** in practice instead of talking about what **we could do**. One of the things that we could not do was promote and sell nutritional supplements in our office.

The logic of this law escaped me, since people who knew nothing about nutrition were legally allowed to sell supplements. On the other hand, I had considerable knowledge about nutrition but risked the loss of my license if I discussed this essential aspect of natural healing with my patients. Rebel that I am, I often talked about nutrition anyway. At the same time, I was active in chiropractic state politics trying to get this law changed. Eventually, in the year 2002, the law was finally amended to include nutrition.

During those early years of nutrition work, I made an arrangement with a local health food store to carry many of the supplements that I regularly recommended to my patients. In this way, if any authority challenged me over making nutritional recommendations, at least I was in the defensible position of honestly stating that I was not making a profit from their sale.

Also during those years, once again at the recommendation of Dr. Meed West, I attended a new type of muscle response testing seminar that I found much more user-friendly than Applied Kinesiology. It was called "Contact Reflex Analysis" (CRA), developed and taught by Dr. D.A. Versendaal. Having been a student of AK developer Dr. Goodheart, Dr. Versendaal's technique used only a single strong muscle and primarily utilized *electrical points* in the body, called "contact reflexes". As a rule, these were acupuncture points of the various organs of the body (Versendaal-Hoezee).

I was attracted to this technique because of its efficiency in revealing information from the nervous system in a very short period of time. I credit Dr. Versendaal's work with renewing my interest in specific whole food nutrition therapy, as well as with the marked improvement in my overall health that occurred in the years that I was utilizing CRA. Dr. Versendaal showed me that the path to my own health improvement was truly connected to what I put in my mouth.

In clinical practice, I experienced many successes using CRA, but there was a problem with *consistency* of improvement. For each person who got better with their nutritional program, there was another person who did not. This bothered me a great deal because I knew I was still missing something, but I did not know what it was. But getting great part-time results was much better than not getting results of all, so I continued with CRA until I discovered a new concept.

The next nutrition method I acquired was taught by Dietrich Klinghardt M.D. and later by Freddie Ulan, D.C., called Autonomic Response Technique (ART). The thing I found remarkable about ART was that it acknowledged that all things in the universe had a unique "resonance" or energy signature, based upon the work of Dr. Yoshiaki Omura, a medical doctor from Tokyo, Japan (Klinghardt).

ART also acknowledged that certain toxic substances in the environment could *block* the autonomic nervous system *response*. Immediately, I became interested in this concept because of my experience with CRA; some people would improve and some people would not. Dr. Klinghardt joined with a few other providers, including Dr. Armand DeFelice, DDS, in acknowledging the effect of scarring on the energy of the body. Rather than using acupuncture points, ART used organ pressure to create the muscle "response". I found this technique to be valuable, and used it for the better part of the next 12 years, as the accuracy of the ART testing procedure was a "quantum leap" ahead of what I had been doing to get consistent results using nutrition.

It wasn't until 2009, when Autumn Smith, N.T.P. suggested using virtual cellular energies in a new testing procedure, that I found anything that worked better than ART. The Morphogenic Field Technique has taken my practice to a new level of efficient and accurate healing. Sara's story is a wonderful example of the power of the MFT to change a complicated, perplexing health crisis into a new lease on life.

Sara's Story

> I first met Dr. Springob in June 2008, but my "story" begins many years before that. I am now a 44 year old woman who has, for as long as I can remember, suffered from a variety of unexplained ailments including, but not limited to extreme lethargy, fatigue and severe digestive issues that seem to have manifested in the bowel. These issues have not only been a concern mentally, they have been very disruptive on a practical level to my daily life. Although my problems

seemed unrelated, I could not help but wonder if they were somehow all connected.

Over several years I made many attempts through my physician to discover the cause of these symptoms as they became more unmanageable as time went on. I was repeatedly dismissed and although it was never said directly to me I felt I was labeled a hypochondriac. My severe gas symptoms were put down to "taking too much air in when I ate, chewing gum and drinking carbonated drinks." I did none of these things and was absolutely convinced that even if I did they would not be identified as the root cause of these very significant problems.

I was referred by chance to Dr. Springob in June 2008 and it truly has been a life changing experience. Before I met him and started witnessing a dramatic improvement in my overall health I was skeptical and cynical of his methods – mostly because I did not really understand them initially. I had been dismissed by the traditional medical community so many times not only without a diagnosis, but without treatment. I was desperate for some relief and some answers. At the first appointment and for the first time ever someone in the medical profession was listening not only to my words, but to my body.

After performing some chiropractic adjustments he explained the various muscle response tests he would perform and what they would reveal. At that time he also explained the role of proper personalized nutrition and after completion of the testing he recommended several nutritional supplements to improve my situation and give me some relief. It became apparent through his testing that he was literally able to sense and feel the inflammation in my bowel and treat it accordingly. Within two weeks I noticed a significant improvement and a reduction in my symptoms. More importantly I finally felt we were treating the cause and not just the symptoms.

Initially my visits to him were regular and frequent as I understood that getting to the root of my long term discomfort was a process that would take time to reveal itself as we resolved the various issues. After some time we discovered what I believe to be the major underlying cause of all my health related problems – metal toxicity and in particular lead poisoning. This is the explanation and the "breakthrough" I had been seeking for so long.

Dr. Springob discovered that my body was literally "saturated" and high levels of lead were revealed in my blood, bones, all major organs and even my spinal cord. He advised it would take three to four years to "detoxify". I was shocked, but relieved to know we had made such an important discovery. His analysis proved to be accurate. Now, three years later my symptoms of chronic digestive issues have almost disappeared and occur only on the rare occasion.

I believe the relief I have experienced has been as a result of giving my system what it needs nutritionally to heal itself. I had suspected my difficulties were somehow related to diet, but no specific food allergies had ever been identified so I was unable to make progress without the valuable information discovered through Dr. Springob's testing. I cannot express the relief I feel at my overall good health. My only regret is that I did not find it earlier!

Chapter 6

The Morphogenic Field Technique® Story

"The physician should not treat the disease but the patient who is suffering from it."

-Maimonides

In the fall of 2004, we were looking for a new part-time receptionist to work the evening shift at our clinic. My wife Linda, also the clinic manager, hired a 15 year old high school student named Autumn Smith for the after school job. Autumn took to her new position with ease. She was accurate, efficient, had great people skills and was very happy to be involved with her new routine for a few hours a day.

My first impression of Autumn was that she was a bit malnourished. Even though she stood approximately 5 foot, 6 inches tall, she weighed less than 100 pounds. It wasn't long before I took an interest in her dietary habits and began treating and nutritionally testing her. As a staff member, she was interested in the nutritional aspects of our wellness practice. She expressed curiosity about nutritional healing, and her overall health improved as she implemented much of the nutritional advice I gave her.

Early in her career at our clinic, Autumn became completely supportive of the philosophy of our wellness center. She was attentive and enjoyed listening in on the nutritional education that I provided to patients. In conversation, Autumn had a unique ability to recall and repeat back much of the nutritionally-oriented statements she overheard.

In those days, I often needed assistance from a staff person when performing muscle testing procedures. Prior to the development of the Morphogenic Field Technique®, I found muscle response testing to be quite exhausting. With muscle testing, an energy transfer occurs between practitioner and patient, and this transfer often left me feeling worn out by the end of a long day. The assistance from an *indirect tester* allowed for the completion of an *energy circuit* between the patient, the assistant, and me. I found that using the indirect tester's arm, rather than the patient's, provided a more efficient method of receiving information from the nervous system, and spared me from the otherwise inevitable depletion of my own energy.

Autumn frequently served as the indirect tester, and gradually she increased her exposure to nutrition and energy healing. The longer Autumn worked in our office, the healthier she became. Over time, she added some weight to her frame and she began looking much less pale. We often got into discussions about how her eating habits had changed over time. I was appalled when she told me that while growing up, she had considered Cup o' Noodles to be the perfect food: always available, tasty and easy to prepare. Frozen pizza and Pop Tarts were mainstays, while drinking water was foreign; her favorite beverage had been Kool Aid. To me, this explained a lot about why she had been so pale and anemic when she first came to work for us. As the years went on, Autumn repeatedly expressed a desire for a career in nutritional healing and asked for my help in finding the path to make this possible. Four years after first coming to work in our clinic, Autumn enrolled in Nutritional Therapist training.

My wife Linda, who had worked as the clinic manager for over thirty years, also began to become more involved in the clinical aspects of our busy Wellness Center. She had witnessed many dramatic health improvements over the years and knew well the power of sound nutrition to heal the body. Our children were raised and she was ready for a new challenge, so together, Linda and Autumn took the course offered by the Nutritional Therapy Association and they graduated in November 2009.

The "Light Bulb" Moment

One day in the spring of 2009, Autumn was assisting me as an indirect tester while performing our "old style" nutrition test on a patient. During the procedure, she posed the question that would eventually change everything about our work. The Nutritional Therapy training had led her to rethink the familiar muscle testing process. There was a "disconnect" between what she was learning in her training and the actual method in which we gathered nutritional information from the patient.

The "old style" of nutrition testing was not really all that old. At that time, the procedure we were using in our office was based upon Dr. Dietrich Klinghardt's Autonomic Response Technique (ART). I found it to be the most advanced of all of the muscle response testing procedures available back then. Operating from the premise that a slight manual pressure against *organ reflexes* would cause a *response* from the autonomic nervous system, ART could reveal if that organ was "challenged" in performing its normal function. Consistent with all of the muscle testing techniques I had learned, the *response* would be a weakening of the *locked* test muscle.

Dr. Klinghardt's system involved a process of *matching the resonant energy* of various substances with the resonance of the *responding* organ, and then looking for nutritional ways to *eliminate*, and thus normalize, the response. In this way, ART guided us to the nutritional support that the patient needed to repair that organ.

Everyone in our office was trained, or scripted, to explain ART to patients who asked questions about how it worked. The staff, including myself, had not questioned whether there might be a better method for nutritional testing, until that spring day in 2009. As we were looking for the right combination of whole food nutritional supplements for an *organ response* on a patient, Autumn made her inspired statement regarding testing *cell energies* instead of *organ energies*: "Wouldn't it be better to talk to the cells?"

As the most basic unit of tissue, cells would be a more direct source of information about what the body needs. I was immediately struck by the brilliance of the question. It was the type of out-of-the-box thinking that I had come to expect from Autumn. My response to the question was immediate. "Of course that would be more logical! But how would you do that?" Autumn was one step ahead of me, and she suggested that we call on our mutual friend, Dr. Nick Lamothe, the well-known master of the virtual energy vial.

The Virtual Energy Vials

The *virtual cellular energies* to which Autumn referred are *digitally-created* energies, produced by a unique computer program. They elicit a direct response from the Autonomic Nervous System (ANS) through the interaction with the Morphogenic Field. Although the M-Field is not "hard-wired" like the actual nerves, it is our contention that it can be considered an electromagnetic extension of the ANS. As such, the M-Field reacts through the known channels of nerve communication to the muscles, which respond in a manner that we can measure and interpret.

When these virtual energies are created by Dr. Lamothe, the process is similar to that of video recording. Just as a video camera digitally captures exact images, sounds, and movements and records them on a DVD, the computer program captures the energy signature of various substances and "records" them into vials. The bio-energetic transfer process used to make the vials replicates the resonance, or energy signature, of whatever molecular arrangement you wish to copy.

Autumn's idea was to acquire a *copy of the virtual energy of the cells,* and then use the virtual energy to elicit an informative response from the Morphogenic Field. Thus began the weird and wondrous journey that led us to the creation of *Morphogenic Field Technique (MFT)* and *M-Field Signature Matching.*

Autumn's insistence and perseverance finally led me to the telephone. I made a personal phone call to Dr. Lamothe and told him what we were looking for. After a brief conversation, he agreed to send me the vials of 50 types of cellular virtual energies. They arrived a few days later and we began to experiment to see what effect they would have on a muscle response test. We were not prepared for what followed. The body energy that we had been working with was suddenly amplified in a way that made it easier to feel, understand, and respond to.

The "Old-Style" Energy Drain

Similar to other professional competencies, it is not unusual for people who practice muscle response testing for many years to develop a type of "sixth-sense"; an ability to sense the energy field of healthy people. For healers who practice the various types of muscle response testing, a long day of treating and testing sick people can be extremely draining. We might wish to help everyone, but energy conservation and self-preservation are crucial, and this energy drain affects the ability to practice for long hours.

Awareness of this energy depletion motivated us to find a way to objectively measure the torus energy, or, the M-Field. We observed that the energy would often change as the virtual energy test kits were brought toward the patient. This reaction would occur several inches or even feet away from the corporeal body. We were intrigued by this phenomenon and began looking for a consistent way to test it and quantify it. One day, we formulated an idea that made quantifying the size of the body's energy field easy, accurate and reproducible.

Standard Process®, the organic whole food nutritional supplement company manufactures two nutritional supplements to support the hormone systems of the body: Symplex® M, for the male endocrine system, and Symplex® F, for the female endocrine system. We accurately reasoned that the energy field of the body should automatically reject the energy signature of a supplement designed for the opposite gender. In other words, a woman's energy field should reject Symplex® M and the man's energy field should reject Symplex® F.

We tested our hypothesis by performing a modified muscle response test. Just as predicted, when the Symplex® M supplement came in contact with the *boundary* of Autumn's energy field, the test muscle dramatically weakened. On that particular day, the boundary of Autumn's energy field measured approximately 2 feet from her corporeal body. We then reversed the procedure. Using the female endocrine supplement Symplex® F, Autumn duplicated the same modified muscle response test on my energy field with similar results: my body did not want the female hormone support.

Our next step was to determine if the right nutritional solutions could increase the "size" of the M-Field measurement. Following an old style nutritionally-based muscle response test, Autumn ingested the supplement that her body showed a positive response to. Then, we re-measured her field by repeating the modified muscle response test with the Symplex® M to find the new boundary of Autumn's energy field. After ingesting the supplement, her *energy field had more than doubled in size to over 4 feet*!

Again we reversed the procedure, this time with Autumn testing me, and again, the results were similar. After that, we had a new working hypothesis: providing the correct nutritional supplementation could increase the output of a person's energy signature, and therefore, increase the size of their M-field.

Morphogenic Field Testing is Born

Over time, working with patients in the everyday practice, we began every testing procedure by measuring the dimensions of what we came to call the Morphogenic Field or M-Field. We consistently found that people with a small or asymmetrical M-Field were *challenged* in their ability to heal. Conversely, we found that people with large, balanced M-Fields consistently had fewer symptoms and healed faster. This simple concept would be the key to additional progress in the world of muscle response testing for nutritional deficiencies.

As we searched for a name for our new-found technique, we considered three or four different types of nomenclature. The first name that we tried was "Cellular Communication Technique". Essentially, the name was appropriate since our intention was to communicate with the cells. In fact, we went so far as to purchase the web domain name <u>www. cellularcommunicationtechnique.com</u>. But that was as far as it went.

The real inspiration for the name Morphogenic Field Technique (MFT) can be attributed to synchronicity. Dr. Royal Lee, the founder of the organic whole food supplement company Standard Process, Inc. had written a paper in the late 1940s describing Protomorphogens™ and their role in cellular function. I had been reviewing the details of that paper, looking for nutritional concepts that should be included in our new procedure designed to provide optimum cellular communication and nutrition.

Dr. Lee's Protomorphogen™ theory spoke of the need for *cellular blueprints* during the break down of older cells and the growth of new cells. Wishing to address all aspects of cellular construction in MFT, we included Protomorphogen™ supplementation protocols into every nutritional program we designed.

In addition to the discussion of cellular blueprints, Dr. Lee's Protomorphogen™ paper emphasized the somewhat nebulous concept of a *Morphinogenic Field*, an energy field that would somehow direct the cellular degeneration and regeneration process. It reminded me of some of Dr. Albert Einstein's early references to universal energy fields. Einstein proposed that a form of energy exists between the known atomic particles; a type of unseen control mechanism that directs the quantum mechanics.

It seems both of these great men of science were referring to the same life energy, and their theories resonated with my belief in the concept of Innate Intelligence. I consulted with Autumn and we agreed to name our technique after this *field of energy that ultimately directs the most important life processes*. In the word *morphogenic*, "morph" implies change; "genic" implies origination. This word was in keeping with our goal of originating change at the cellular level through communication with the body's energy field. Even with a name that fit perfectly, it took us approximately one year to put it all together.

Chapter 7

The Development of the Morphogenic Proteins

"I have had my results for a long time: but I do not yet know how I am to arrive at them."

-Karl Friedrich Gauss

When the first batch of vials arrived from Nick's office, our goal was to assess whether or not the introduction of virtual cellular energy changed our ability to draw *information* from the Morphogenic Field. These new vials created a much greater energy effect than what we originally anticipated. The simple introduction of these vials to the M-Field was enough to objectively enhance the field energy as measured using Symplex® M or Symplex ®F.

We spent many hours using these 50 vials in various ways, looking for the combinations that would create the largest energy affect. As we continued through this experimentation process, it became clear that we needed to create a test kit specifically designed to gain maximum energetic information from the cells. So in November of 2009, right after Linda and Autumn graduated from Nutritional Therapy school, we all paid a visit to the office of Dr. Nick Lamothe.

By the time we visited Nick, we were using the M-Field almost exclusively in our testing procedure at the office. Nick listened as we laid-out our plan. We were interested in the dietary factors that were not being adequately addressed by other muscle response testing systems; specifically the concepts of *foundational nutrition* and *toxicity*. *Foundational nutrition* refers to the nutrients that all cells need for proper growth and reproduction, whereas *toxicity* represents the presence of unwanted, harmful substances. With Nick's help, we hoped to create virtual energy test kits that would identify foundational nutritional deficiencies and the presence of toxic energies as part of a routine assessment.

Firmly convinced of the power of the vials to elicit helpful information from the energy field, our priority became the creation of a comprehensive testing kit of cellular energies. We considered our options from among what seemed to be infinite possibilities, and eventually requested a total of 190 virtual energies of the nucleic proteins from various cells.

Nick was enthusiastic and is highly capable, and within a few days, the 190 cellular virtual energies arrived at our office. The sheer number presented a hindrance to the creation of a workable system, which needed to fit into one usable test kit of 60 vials or less. Knowing that we needed to trim down the number of energies, we began combining (or layering) individual energies to maximize their analytical effect. The plan was to combine compatible energies together into fewer single vials. Experience had shown us that adding one synergistic vial to another gave us more accurate readings.

We spent the next two weekends systematically and methodically categorizing the vials according to their cellular function. Then, we set about the long process of "matching-up" the energies. We found, for example, that all the *joint-related energies* could be combined into one vial that included the nucleic protein resonance from the cells of cartilage, tendons, ligaments, synovial membranes and intervertebral discs.

There were some surprises along the way. For instance, while there was only one vial for the 10 joint-related energies, the blood-related nucleic proteins required eight separate vials because none of these energies were attuned with each other. At the end of our two week project, we had narrowed the 190 nucleic protein energies into 58 compatible vials.

Collectively, we named them the Morphogenic Proteins. We then labeled the combination vials according to their *energetic contents*. Normal nucleic protein energies were abbreviated NP (normal proteins) while the aberrant energies were called SNP (support proteins). Some of the Morphogenic Protein vials contained only NP energies, others only SNP energies, and some were combinations.

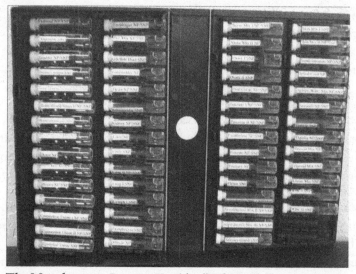

The Morphogenic Protein Kit (the "White Kit") contains the energy of 190 different cells that can be found in the human body.

When we had completed our first MFT Test Kit, we immediately began using this kit as a replacement for the old-style body scan to identify which cells of the body were requesting nutritional attention. A dysfunction in the body will usually manifest as an aberrant energy when introduced to the Morphogenic Proteins. The MP Kit identifies the body's M-Field response to an individual cellular energy vial in the kit. In this way, the M-Field response to the vials in the Morphogenic Protein kit replaced the body scan. It is what differentiates MFT from any other muscle response technique.

The advantages of using this kit were immediately obvious. First, even when performed without the assistance of an indirect tester, the energy drain that I had always experienced was eliminated. Secondly, the information obtained was suddenly more comprehensive and much easier to classify. Since information is the basis for all future action, quicker analysis led to quicker action.

Every time we found an "attraction" to one of the Morphogenic Proteins, we removed the vial from the test kit and had the patient hold it. This step of putting the vial *in-the-field* created an additional energy affect that allowed us to find problems that were previously hidden. Our experimentation continued to reveal new possibilities. We discovered that adding one energy to another often increased the size of the M-Field. Every time we increased the size of the M-Field, the test kits became more sensitive. We used the term "energy layering" to describe this phenomenon. During this phase of development, it seemed every day was a new adventure of discovery.

As our patients became accustomed to the new testing procedure, one of the most common, yet unexpected, comments was that the new style of testing felt less intrusive than our previous methods. I was pleased to hear that patients were more comfortable with our new M-Field testing technique where the *vials* do the differentiation for us. Although we made many changes to the test kits that we developed later in the process, we have yet to alter the Morphogenic Protein Test Kit. We got this one right the first time!

The Cellular Construction Project

When we were satisfied with the Morphogenic Protein Test Kit, we began to work on the *Foundations Test Kit*. In our work at Boulevard Natural Wellness Center, we are constantly reminded of how the American diet in its present state is far from complete. As Weston Price found when he did his studies of primitive societies, the nutrient value of our current food supply is a small fraction of that of our ancestors. This could be viewed in a positive light, since our bodies have the unique ability to glean nutrition from even the worst diet. However, we are all too familiar with the problems that result. The evidence is undeniable that giving the body wholesome, nutrient-dense food is a much more desirable option.

In MFT, we approach Foundational Nutrition from the perspective of a "cellular construction project". If you made the decision today to build a new house, you would be looking at a project that would take at least six months to complete, start to finish. At this very moment, without you even thinking about it, there is a huge construction project going in your body. In the next 24 hours, your body will be constructing somewhere between *30 billion to 60 billion new cells*.

Tomorrow, you will do it all again…and the next day… and every day after that. Do any of us have what it takes to complete this huge task?

Let's hope so, because it's going to happen whether we are ready or not! As time goes by, those cells will get together and make new tissues, then those tissues will replace the organs that are now functioning. It is a constantly renewing, dynamic system, and the good news is, every day we have the chance to make it better.

The cellular construction project is similar to the construction of a house. To build a house, you need three things in order to start: a clean construction site, quality building materials, and blueprints to guide the process.

Most people would never consider building their new home at the city dump. When Linda and I built a new house several years ago, we looked for a lot that was clear of debris, stable and equipped to make the best possible place for our new home. The MFT Foundations Test Kit functions similarly, as it identifies the presence of the energy of various toxins within the body, a sort of *quality control* for cellular construction. In other words, the Foundations Test Kit screens the M-Field to make sure the construction site is clean.

Next in the construction of our house, Linda and I needed access to building materials, preferably the best ones available. Just as the construction of a building requires appropriate materials, the construction of a healthy cell requires the highest quality organic whole food. The nutritional supplement energies in the Foundation Kit represent the raw materials needed to build a healthy cell. Whether in our homes or in our bodies, we should not settle for faulty building materials. The Foundations Kit indicates which materials are needed during the body's current phase of construction.

Our son Matthew is a commercial journeyman electrician. He says that he can always tell how well the construction project will turn out based upon how many sets of blueprints are available. If the workers have to walk across the construction site to check the blueprints, there will be times when this extra step seems burdensome and the workers look for short-cuts. That is how mistakes are made. Heeding Matthew's advice, Linda and I made sure each of the laborers working on our house had their own set of blueprints to refer to as they worked.

Cells have blueprints as well, called Protomorphogens™ (PMG). In his ground-breaking research paper, *An Introduction to Protomorphology*™, Dr. Royal Lee described the PMG as, "that component of the cell chromosome that is responsible for the morphinogenetic determination of cell characteristics." Blueprints are essential; therefore the Foundations Kit works to verify that there are enough on site to get the job done right.

Without a clean building site, high-quality materials, and a generous supply of PMG's, the new cells will be of poor quality. This means that the tissues will also be poor quality and ultimately, the whole body will be poor quality. The cellular construction project continues throughout our lifespan, and since we are going to be building cells no matter what we do, we might as well make the best ones that we can. After all, our future health depends upon it.

Let's Build a Cell

In addition to the basics for construction, all cells need proper hydration. If water can be considered a nutrient, it is the most important one. The chemical formula, H_2O, illustrates the incredible number of tasks that water performs. Two positively charged hydrogen ions are balanced by one oxygen ion, which is negatively charged. The resulting electrical nature of water helps maintain normal energetic flow in the body to facilitate communication between the cells. In the MFT Energy Signature Matching technique, cell-to-cell communication is of the utmost importance for accuracy of the information we gather from the M-Field.

It is common knowledge that while human beings cannot live more than a few days without this essential nutrient, which is second only to oxygen in terms of its importance to survival. However, even when we have enough to *get by*, low-grade dehydration can cause all sorts of problems. Water plays a role in the regulation of body temperature. Many times I have encountered patients who complained of feeling either chilled or feverish, when the actual problem was dehydration. This seems to occur more in the winter, when the body's signals are more likely to be interpreted as hunger rather than thirst. In the summertime, sunshine and heat prompt most of us acknowledge our thirst and quench it by drinking water.

Dr. Frank Springob

Water removes wastes and toxins from the body. The lymphatic system functions much like a municipal sewer system. The cells give off waste products during routine metabolism which is carried by the lymphatics toward the general direction of the kidneys. The kidneys are comparable to the sewage treatment plant, where the metabolic toxins are eliminated from the body through the urine. If the kidneys do not have sufficient water, the urine becomes concentrated, which causes problems in both the short and the long term.

In addition to removing waste, water also provides oxygen to the cells. Water is the main component of the blood, which carries oxygen to all the tissues of the body. It also acts as a shock absorber for both the joints and the organs. Without the *cushioning* provided by sufficient hydration, normal everyday movements can become unnecessarily painful.

This is the short list. Some people have written entire books on the importance of drinking sufficient amounts of pure, clean water on a daily basis. Water makes up about 60% of our total body mass, and it is required for every chemical reaction that takes place in the body. Many of the beverages that Americans consume daily have a *diuretic* effect in the body, meaning the drink removes more water than it replaces. Such is the case with coffee, soda and teas with caffeine. Ideally, we should drink about one half of our body weight in ounces of water per day. In advising my patients, I limit this to a total of 100 ounces of water per day; drinking more than that risks the possibility of washing-out too many electrolytes from the system.

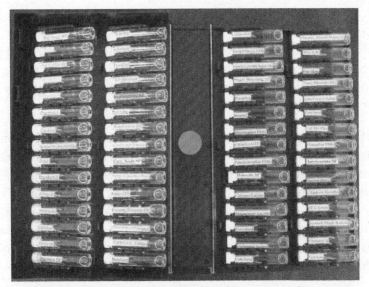

The MFT Foundations kit (the "Red Kit") contains the energies of substances that all cells need for healthy growth and reproduction.

When using the MFT Foundations Kit, hydration is the first detail we test for. If the Foundations Kit indicates a problem in this area, we must first rule out if the person is drinking enough water. If a sufficient amount of water is being consumed, then we consider if there are any biochemical imbalances in the body which mimic dehydration. There are several conditions that can contribute to this type of situation.

For example, electromagnetic field (EMF) sensitivity sometimes manifests itself in symptoms of dehydration. We are all constantly bombarded by stray EMF's in our modern world. Sources include cell phones, high-voltage power lines, computers, microwave ovens and fluorescent lights. While they vary in intensity and proximity to the body, every electrical device puts off an electromagnetic field. Given the electrical nature of water, it is not surprising that EMF's can have this kind of impact.

B-vitamin deficiencies can also create problems with water balance, including retention and absorption challenges. B-vitamins are a family of nutrients which must be balanced in the body. Briefly stated, the deficiency of vitamin B6 tends to create an imbalance wherein the cells retain water. Additionally, a deficiency of niacinamide, another part of the B-vitamin family, will prevent the cells from absorbing water efficiently. The proper whole food B-vitamin supplement will rebalance the situation.

Clinically, we have observed that people with high uric acid also have difficulty with healthy fluid transfer in their tissues. Energetically, this can also present as a form of dehydration which can often be resolved with the proper whole food nutritional supplement. I have worked with many patients who, after added nutritional support, return to my office with a report of lowered uric acid in their latest blood test.

All of these potential problems are addressed as part of the routine Foundational Testing Procedure. They are included in the area of hydration because of the effect they can have on the body's use of water. When considering the role of quality food and pure water in providing the ideal environment for cellular construction, the difference of optimal nutrition amounts to the difference between weak cells and healthy cells, between *merely surviving* and *thriving*. The goal of Morphogenic Field Technique is to help everyone find what their body needs to *thrive*.

Chapter 8

The Foundational Role of Proper Digestion

"If we are what we eat, with all the genetically modified and imitation foods, what the heck are we?"

~Unknown

We have all heard the old saying, "you are what to eat." Although this is accurate, the hidden truth behind this proverb is that you actually, "are what you can digest and absorb." It is not only important to eat foods that are nutrient-dense; you must then place yourself in a relaxed environment during meals, chew your food properly and allow your balanced autonomic nervous system to do the rest.

In my opinion, the greatest marketing scams of all time are the commercials that tell us the reason we have heartburn is the presence of excess stomach acid. Nothing could be further from the truth. Hypochlorhydria, insufficient stomach acid, is a much more common condition than *excess* acid. The fact is, most heartburn is a result of eating *the wrong foods in the wrong places in the wrong way.* If we were all properly chewing only organic, whole food in a calm, happy environment, there would be very little heartburn for us to talk about.

Wrong Food, Wrong Place, Wrong Time

Over the last 100 years, we have been eating increasing amounts of hydrogenated and trans fats. The body cannot process these fats in the same way it does the fats that the natural world provides. Hydrogenated fat is artificial, harmful, and heavily marketed to convince us that it is perfectly fine for us to consume it. Even the mainstream medical establishment acknowledges that eating hydrogenated fat increases the risk of heart disease, stroke, and type 2 diabetes. Our bodies are unable to digest this manufactured substance, which leads to higher levels of liver stress and gall bladder disease due to the *sludgy bile* that it creates. Improper fat digestion is one of the main causes of heartburn, and the problem is now chronic, as these fats are ever-present on American grocery store shelves.

Also in the group of "wrong foods" is sugar. Consider that refined sugar did not even exist until 400 years ago. Now, it is everywhere in copious amounts. I tell patients that the recipe for heartburn is to combine wheat and sugar together; they are like nitro and glycerin to create a "gut bomb". Although the average American has begun to cut back on their sugar intake, we still consume over 100 pounds of refined sugar per person every year. The worst offender in the sugar group is high fructose corn syrup, a highly-processed unnatural sugar made from corn that is now present in almost all of our industrial foods. In performing the MFT *energy signature matching* procedure, every person tested with high fructose corn syrup reacts negatively to it.

Finally, much of our food now is consumed *on the run*. Digestion is a *parasympathetic* function; it is meant to occur when we are calm and relaxed. The busy, hectic American lifestyle has made it necessary for us to eat fast-food, and eat it *fast*. Chain restaurants are notorious for obtaining food as a *commodity*, because it is not the quality of the food, but the profit, that is their top priority. It helps to keep in mind that *food* and *food products* are not one and the same. Even the process of preparing a meal starts the early stages of digestion; as we cut those vegetables or beat those eggs, our senses are stimulated and our thoughts turn towards anticipation. In the body-mind, we become primed to digest our food and get the most out of that meal. Microwaving a frozen pot pie short circuits this process and robs us, both nutritionally and psychologically, of the satisfaction of a nourishing meal.

A Synopsis of Digestion

Let's assume there is a *highly unusual* person who follows all the rules of eating properly. They are consuming high quality nutrient-dense food in a happy, restful environment and chewing properly. What are the digestive considerations beyond this point? The three general regions that must be functioning well for proper digestion are the stomach, the small intestine/pancreas, and the liver/gall bladder.

Properly digested nutrients are the building blocks of cellular construction. In order to build a healthy cell, both macronutrients and micronutrients are needed. It is safe to say that if the digestion of the macronutrients is done efficiently, the micronutrients will take care of themselves, provided they are present in the food in the first place.

Macronutrients are complex carbohydrates, fats and protein, each of which requires a two-step process for digestion. With the exception of fats, each process begins in one part of the digestive tract and concludes in another. For example, complex carbohydrates begin breaking down the moment they are chewed, which is one of reasons that proper chewing is so important to efficient digestion.

The complex carbohydrates begin to break down as the teeth mechanically grind the food. Saliva contains an enzyme called amylase which further converts the complex carbohydrates into simple carbohydrates, our main source of immediate fuel. Later in the process, the digestion of the remaining complex carbohydrates will be completed by additional amylase produced by the pancreas. This progression begins in the mouth and is finished in the small intestine, thanks to pancreatic enzymes.

The digestion of protein begins primarily in the stomach. Although there is some mechanical breakdown of the protein due to chewing, it is the hydrochloric acid in the stomach that begins to split apart the complete protein into individualized amino acids. The amino acids of the protein consumed will later be reassembled by your body to create "you." Again, this two-step process is finished in the small intestine after a contribution of proteolytic enzymes from the pancreas.

In the case of fat, the process is delayed. The large fat globules in the food begin to be broken-down by bile, which originates from the liver but is stored in the gallbladder until needed. Once again, this is a two-step process. The bile emulsifies, or breaks down the large fat globules into smaller fat globules, and then the process can be finished by the pancreatic enzyme lipase. If there is insufficient bile to break down the large globules, fat digestion remains incomplete. The pancreatic lipase alone is not sufficient to breakdown the fat all by itself.

Finding the Digestive Problem

All of these processes must take place efficiently and thoroughly to enjoy complete and asymptomatic digestion. If food is eaten and digested properly, a person should be almost totally unaware of the digestion processes taking place. Some people who are reading this and have issues with digestion may already be able to recognize the origin of their symptoms just from this short synopsis. However, most people need to seek out professional help to get to the root cause of their problem.

When patients come into my office complaining of symptoms such as gas, bloating, belching, heartburn or sharp pain either before or after eating, the Foundations Kit often reveals an attraction to the energies of these digestive processes. The Morphogenic Field Technique testing procedure can quickly and efficiently identify the weak link in the chain. In priority order, each of these three systems is tested, looking for both weaknesses and solutions. The Digestion I vials identify imbalances in the pH, or acid balance of the stomach, while the Digestion II vials test for energetic imbalances in the enzyme phases of digestion. Finally, the Digestion III vials test energetically for issues relating to the phases of fat digestion. Once the problem area is understood, we can energetically identify possible solutions, which of course will be completely natural and free of unwanted side effects.

Chapter 9

The Effects of Scarring

"It's a shallow life that doesn't give a person a few scars."

~ Garrison Keillor

The next group of vials in the Foundations Kit identifies abnormal energy readings coming from *active scars*. Most people know where their scars are and even have a few interesting stories associated with them. However, what many do not know is that, according to the nervous system, any healed break in the skin is technically a scar. This includes puncture wounds, belly-buttons, vaccination sites, and tattoos, to name a few. Although they are long-healed, these injuries to the skin can still short-circuit the energy flow of the body.

Scars can be responsible for a phenomenon called "switching". First described by Dr. George Goodheart, *switching* can result in a situation where proper nutritional therapy becomes ineffective. This is due to the neurological confusion created by the abnormal energy of an "active" scar.

Briefly, the energy of the nervous system, which runs all body processes, becomes confused when the signal returning to the brain from a scarred area contains *inaccurate information*. The brain cannot discern these *abnormal readings* from the normal feedback that it regularly receives from the unscarred areas of the body. So, the signal sent by the scarred area *to the brain* may generate an inaccurate response *from the brain*. This causes the *switching*, and it ultimately creates the wrong physiological result.

Fortunately, this only seems to happen in about ten percent of the cases. But for those ten percent, health improvement will be in jeopardy unless the practitioner can recognize the problem and provide the proper solution. For this reason, *Scar Energies* are addressed at this point in the Foundational Testing Procedure, to be ruled out or resolved before we proceed further.

To determine whether a scar is actively interfering with the M-Field, we rely on an informal rubric of decision making. Aside from visual evidence of scars or patient reports which suggest switching, the MFT *Scarring* vial may yield an attraction to the body, as indicated by a strong test muscle. When this happens, it is time to go on a "scar search". For this, we use a variant of the Contact Reflex Analysis technique of Dr. D.A. Versendaal call the *Pulsing Procedure* over an active scar.

MFT defines an *active* scar as a healed break on the skin that is *not "pulsing" at a normal level of energy*. For most of the body, the normal *pulse* over the skin will be a 10. To quantify the pulse over a scar, the practitioner needs to touch the scar in question with one hand, while lightly "pumping" the locked test muscle with the other hand and counting each pump. So, in other words, if I was testing a scar, I might touch the scarred area with my left hand and pump the patient's locked muscle with my right hand. With each pump I would count: 1,2,3,4, and so on. If the energy of the scar is normal, the test muscle will lose its lock at the count of 10. If the muscle loses its lock at any number other than 10, I conclude there is an *aberrant energy* associated with that scar. Scars are inconsistent in the manner in which they disrupt the energy flow; some wreak havoc frequently, others rarely. Fortunately, the treatment for them all is quick and simple.

In treating scars, the two primary tools used to normalize the aberrant energies are *wheat germ oil* and *cold laser energy*. In up to 90% of cases, the deviant scar energy can be eliminated by one or both of these modalities. Both solutions are represented in the Foundations Kit vials, and whichever one attracts to the M-Field is administered to the patient **immediately** so that the Energy Signature Matching process can continue efficiently and accurately.

A video demonstrating of the handling of an active scar can be viewed by visiting the MFT website at www.m-field.info.

Chapter 10

Fat: The Misunderstood Macronutrient

Let food be your medicine and medicine be your food.

~Hippocrates

Recently, I was listening to a local television health news program that ran a segment on the subject of eating fat. This newscast, meant to inform the public, was filled with reams of misinformation. Toeing the party line of the commercial food industry that "all fats are equal", the announcer made no differentiation between natural, healthy sources of fat and the poisonous hydrogenated and trans-fats we have been eating in this country for the last hundred years.

With many sources of factual information available, these news organizations still rely on the *disinformation* (information intentionally meant to confuse the public) that is supplied by the large food conglomerates. The cynical side of me tends to correlate the *disinformation* to the fact that food and drug companies are the manufacturers of these phony-fats, and also tend to be recurring sponsors of these news shows.

The newscast was correct in recommending total fat intake be kept at reasonable levels, and around 30 percent of total calories is a good measure. However, in this age of abundant, fabricated, food-type products, the *quantity* of the fat is a secondary consideration to the *source* of fat.

Here is the truth about fat: Not only are natural fats absolutely necessary for total health, they have many other benefits. Fat is the body's primary source of long-term energy. If carbohydrates are akin to the paper you use to start a fire, then fat is the log you put on the fire to keep it burning. Fat serves as a protective lining for the internal organs; without it, we are more vulnerable to traumatically induced internal injuries. A deficiency or imbalance of proper fatty acids can also lead to fundamental weakness in the cell membranes.

Many people do not know that the fat content of food regulates the rate of nutrient absorption in the small intestine. It also acts as a dampener for blood sugar, slowing the spike that goes along with eating high-glycemic foods. Additionally, natural fat is the only source for the essential fat-soluble vitamins A, D, E, and K. Therefore, a lack of dietary fat can lead to a wide range deficiencies resulting in a wide range of problems.

And finally, it is the fat content of the food that makes it taste good. There are many snacks on the market that are declared to be "low-fat" or "fat-free", and supposedly, a healthier option. The manufacturers hawk these products under names like "Healthy Choice" and "Sensible Sweets", but to make the food taste better, they have substituted the fat with extra sugar or chemical sweeteners. It makes one wonder what exactly it is about this nutrition strategy that is either "healthy" or "sensible"?

Good Fats Verses Bad Fats

In the early 1920's, a young medical internist named Paul Dudley White introduced a great new tool to his colleagues at Harvard. His machine, the electrocardiograph, could reveal the presence of arterial blockage for early diagnosis of heart disease. However, in those days heart disease was rare, and it is rumored that his fellow doctors could imagine few opportunities to use such a device, and so advised him to find a more profitable branch of medicine.

Over the next three decades, something shifted. By the mid 1950's, heart disease had become the leading cause of death in America! Though once uncommon, heart disease remains the number one killer, and according to the CDC, the financial impact of cardiovascular disease reaches into the $400 billion range annually. We might ask ourselves, "How did we get here?" The answer can be found in the disinformation that is propagated nationwide.

Heart disease in the United States began at the time when the major food companies first altered the fats in processed food. There was a dramatic rise in coronary artery disease within 10 years of the introduction of hydrogenated vegetable oil in 1910. Crisco went on sale in 1911 and was marketed as a replacement for natural saturated fats. Later, hydrogenated corn oil, cottonseed oil and then margarine were introduced to replace natural butter and lard. Along with these new products, a huge marketing campaign was initiated to convince the public that these fats were superior to natural fats. Americans were led to believe that man-made fats were better than natural fats, and for a while they seemed to be a miracle of science.

Hydrogenated fats extend the shelf life of processed food. They do not spoil. In fact, chemically speaking, margarine has a similar molecular structure to plastic. Microbes are attracted to butter and it becomes rancid when left out at room temperature too long. Crisco, however, could be left out for years and it would remain in its original condition. It gives pause to wonder, if the microbes won't touch it, why should we?

Despite the bad rap that fat has received in recent years, high quality, naturally occurring fat is no threat. In an optimum diet, 30% of our total caloric intake should come from natural fat; the real issue is the source of the fat. The truth is we should be consuming natural fats from a variety of sources to ensure a proper fat ratio. There are three main types of healthy dietary fat included in the ratio: 30% saturated fat, 60% mono-unsaturated fat and 10% polyunsaturated fat.

Although saturated fat has been unfairly demonized as a factor in coronary artery disease, natural sources are healthful. Excellent sources of saturated fat include butter, coconut oil, palm oil, eggs, raw dairy and meats from pastured and uncaged animals. At 60% of our total fat consumption, mono-unsaturated fat should be among the foods we ingest most frequently. Healthy sources include quality olive oil and the oils found in cashews, almonds, peanuts, pecans and avocados. These oils should be purchased in dark containers and used fairly quickly to prevent them from becoming rancid. Heating this group of oils can damage them, so they are best used on salads or for dipping.

Polyunsaturated fats require more differentiation. Although this group only represents about 10% of the fat ratio, it contains the incredibly important Omega 3 and Omega 6 essential fatty acids. As I am fond of telling my patients, they are called essential fatty acids because they are "essential". We must have these present at all times for total health. Examples include flax oil, fish oil and some of the oils from nuts and seeds. My personal favorite is wheat germ oil and I take it every day. Wheat germ oil is unique in that contains both the omega 3's and the omega 6's. It is also the highest known natural dietary source of the vitamin E complex.

The MFT "Fatty Acid Balancing" Procedure

Toward the end of the Morphogenic Field Technique Testing Procedure, we include a segment that insures that the person being tested has the proper balance of fatty acids. Over the years, many of our most perplexing symptoms were solved by providing the patient with the right type and balance of fats and oils.

For multiple generations, as a population we have been consuming damaging, adulterated hydrogenated/trans fats and believing we were becoming healthier. To the contrary, there is now a great deal of evidence that these man-made fats have contributed significantly to our current national health crisis.

In our Wellness Center, using an energy approach to fatty acid balance, we have witnessed dramatic improvements in patient health and symptomology. Eliminating bad fat is only one piece of the puzzle: they must be replaced by high quality, natural fats. We have had many patients over the years whose complaints were created by low fat diets. Although the dangers of a low fat diet have been publicized recently, there are still many uninformed people who need to learn the truth about the dangers of depriving the body of the fat and oils that it needs to stay healthy.

The Problems With A Low Fat Diet

In 1991, a large, well-known, international company that specializes in weight loss was forced to admit to investors that it faced over 300 pending lawsuits. The suits claimed that the low fat diet recommended by the company was responsible for numerous cases of gallbladder disease. The company was eventually forced to file Chapter 11 bankruptcy in 1993.

This company still exists today, but has now switched focus. Their new claim is that weight loss success is the result of controlling carbohydrates in the diet rather than fat. The company's current stream of commercials imply that weight loss is assured if you buy the food that they prepackage and process, which is designed specifically to parallel their program claims. The commercials provide many "before and after" pictures to prove that it is a formula for success. If this company was wrong in 1991, is it possible they could be wrong again?

The earlier marketing campaign made sense to a lot of people and leads us to wonder, what went wrong with the low fat diet? The answer is simple: Our bodies need fat! No society in history has ever lived on a low fat diet successfully over time. In the 1930's Dr. Weston Price did his extensive studies on the diets of native people from all over the globe. Everywhere he went, he found diets high in natural fats. While the normal fat content of native food averaged about 30% of the intake, there were some variations based on climate. Not surprisingly, the intake was higher in the cooler climates and less in dry, arid climates. The bottom line is the same regardless: no healthy culture has ever been sustained on a low-fat diet.

Bad Fat, or Bad Information?

The consequences of insufficient fat intake are well documented. As the international diet company eventually learned, low fat consumption can lead to gallbladder disease. Dietary fat is necessary to trigger a contraction of the gallbladder. If the bile in the gallbladder is not purged on a regular basis, it can become thick, sludgy and static, and may eventually lead to gall stones.

The popular belief about the relationship of the heart and fats is also distorted. The heart muscle is uniquely designed to run on good fat. People who hold back high quality fats in the diet are causing the heart to suffer unnecessarily. At the cellular level, the skeletal muscles of the body require *fatty acid building blocks* to make strong cell membranes. Insufficient fat causes the muscles to weaken very quickly when subjected to repeated stress. In fact, this is the main premise upon which the Fatty Acid Balancing Procedure is based.

The foods that naturally contain vitamins A, D, E and K all have good fat content. These are the fat soluble vitamins, which require fat in order for them to be properly ingested, digested, and used by the body. Therefore, low fat diets automatically lead to a deficiency in these important fat soluble vitamins. Another consideration is that protein, the "bricks" that build our bodies, cannot be properly utilized without sufficient fat.

In our current culture, we are led to believe that cholesterol is something to be feared, and that dietary fat is responsible for causing high levels of cholesterol. In fact, cholesterol plays an important role in hormone production. The adrenal hormones, used for stress recovery, require sufficient serum cholesterol, and the creation of sex hormones such as progesterone and testosterone also require cholesterol.

Many have heard television commercials promoting medications to address hormone imbalance problems. You may have even seen a commercial for a drug to address low testosterone followed immediately by another drug commercial to address high cholesterol. This is typical pharmaceutical company strategy: persuade consumers that for every health complaint there is a miracle drug, a panacea to make them complete. This is no passive endeavor. The campaigns are aggressive, pervasive, and unrelenting. I once counted the commercials while watching the national evening news to see what percentage was sponsored by the drug industry. The average turned out to be approximately 80%. This drug-deficiency model is effective, too. Americans represent only 5% of the world's population, yet we consume 50% of the world's drug production.

Considering all of the hormone imbalance issues evident in our society, a more natural, holistic perspective is called for. The body is more than the sum of its parts; each process affects the next. One person's tendency toward high serum cholesterol may be related to their body's inability to generate sufficient sex hormones at the gland level. Instead of indicating a need for a cholesterol drug and a synthetic hormone replacement, these problems could be interpreted differently. Since cholesterol is necessary to make testosterone, high levels of cholesterol coupled with low levels of testosterone may suggest a fatty acid imbalance. Cholesterol levels may lower naturally if the testicles are given the necessary nutritional support to use the available cholesterol to manufacture more testosterone. This seems to be the situation in some of the cases we have witnessed, although more in depth study is required to validate this hypothesis.

Insufficient available cholesterol levels may also exist in patients taking statin drugs, further challenging the testicles to create the male hormone.

Could it be that the marketing departments of the pharmaceutical industry have distorted these chemical relationships in the body for the purpose of selling more medications? Pharmaceutical companies stand to profit less when consumers are fully informed.

The "Fat Solution"

From the energetic perspective, fat imbalances can be confirmed quickly and easily by using the correct muscle response testing procedure. The entire MFT Fatty Acid Testing Procedure takes less than one minute to perform by a qualified practitioner. Although it is an advanced procedure, we teach it in the MFT Basic Seminar because it is important to learn early in the nutritional healing timeline.

We have had incredible success with several symptomatic clinical presentations using this simple and easy to perform procedure. For example, there have been many cases of pregnant female patients with a history of miscarriage that have benefited greatly from addressing fatty acid imbalance during the pregnancy. Autumn Smith, MFT co-developer, is an example of this success. Coming from a family with a long history of multiple miscarriages, she personally credits this procedure with the success of her last pregnancy.

For people with arthritic-type symptoms, this procedure has been a blessing. Proper fat consumption and balance is important in preventing inflammatory response. We have had literally hundreds of examples in our Wellness Center of people who have achieved arthritic pain relief from the *fatty acid status* information provided by this simple test. Other patients reported improved musculoskeletal strength and endurance. Additionally, correcting wheat germ oil deficiency has been extremely effective in supporting the oxygenation of the tissues in people with both pulmonary and cardiac symptoms.

I am very proud of the results we have achieved since adding this procedure to the Morphogenic Field Technique. If another procedure exists where a patient's specific fatty acid needs can be identified in less than a minute, we are unaware of it.

Chapter 11

Energy—Where Should We Go To Get Some?

"Carob works on the principle that, when mixed with the right combination of fats and sugar, it can duplicate chocolate in color and texture. Of course, the same can be said of dirt."

-Sandra Boynton

We all know the harsh reality: sugar and fat make everything taste better. But in our quest for something tasty, we often sacrifice more than we know.

In its 16th century beginnings, the sugar trade flourished because of the slave trade. In their book, "Sugar Changed the World", authors Marina Budhos and Marc Aronson describe the demand for sugar as it swept across Europe and the Americas, enabled by the cruel exploitation of African and South Asian people. As sugar became more available to the common man, more output was expected from the factory workers who ate it. The prevalence of sugar satisfied the appetites of both the consumer and the investor, providing immediate energy and increased productivity.

Keeping blood sugar up is still important for good energy. However, as most people know, blood sugar that is elevated too high or for too long causes significant damage to the body. With the advent of new, scientifically developed sweeteners, we now have many options to feed our cravings for both the taste and the rush of sugar. Energy drinks and diet colas have replaced tea with sugar for the midday pick-me-up. However, many of these sugar-alternatives come with their own hidden costs, and we must ask ourselves, how much of a price are we willing to pay?

Because sugar is such a huge problem for so many people, the next priority in the Foundations Kit is labeled *Sugar Handling*. Similar to the subject of fat, sugar cannot be properly evaluated unless we differentiate the type of sugar we are talking about. Sugar comes in many forms; some have nutritional value, most resemble poison to the body.

For our bodies to function on a day-to-day basis, fuel is needed. While fat provides the long term fuel, it is carbohydrates that provide the short-term energy needs of the body. As described in the earlier log-on-the-fire analogy, if paper is your only fuel, you're going to need a lot of it to keep the flame alive.

The organs and glands that are responsible for the carbohydrate/sugar handling process are the pancreas, the liver and the adrenals. To maintain healthy blood sugar levels, the complex carbohydrate breakdown must be a unified effort by the endocrine system; when one component is not working properly, the process is compromised. In a well balanced diet, approximately 40% of the total intake should come from carbohydrates. In the overall mass of the body, carbohydrates make up only about two percent, which means that the carbohydrates eaten today need to be *burned off today* or be stored away for the future.

Whether burned or stored, carbohydrates are converted. At the cellular level, the fuel made from these carbohydrates is called Adenosine-5-triphosphate (ATP). ATP is provided to the cell after a cascade of physiological reactions that lead to the breakdown of complex carbohydrates into simple carbohydrates. When functioning properly, the entire process is extremely methodical. Food sources of complex carbohydrates such as whole grains, legumes and vegetables are digested slowly. When the resulting sugars reach the bloodstream, they are carried to the cells for fuel.

The refined carbohydrates and simple sugars found in sugary foods and energy drinks usurp this route and reach the bloodstream very quickly, challenging the body systems to manage the rapid rise in blood sugar. The temporary quick boost in energy is usually followed by a hypoglycemic crash. Therefore, with the exception of a situation that demands quick energy, the majority of dietary carbohydrates should be in the *complex* form.

An ideal diet and lifestyle, over time, usually leads to a fasting blood sugar level in the range of 70-90 milligrams per deciliter. Sustained higher levels are suspicious and require further investigation to prevent the long-term organ, gland and nerve damage that can result from unrelenting hyperglycemia.

The typical, sugar loaded American diet has created an epidemic of Type II Diabetes, hypertension, and obesity. In the last 200 years, the average American has gone from eating about 5 pounds of refined carbohydrates per year to an estimated 158 pounds per year! The load placed on the pancreas, liver and adrenals by this deluge of sugar has resulted in this frightening fact: the Center for Disease Control (CDC) now estimates that an average American child born in the year 2000 has a one-in-three probability of developing Type II diabetes during their lifetime. Until this alarming trend is reversed, and the sugar addiction is addressed, the financial and human costs will continue to be astronomical.

During the MFT Testing Procedure, the Foundations Kit may energetically identify a response from the M-Field in the area of sugar handling. To interpret this result, the practitioner must next *verbally* inquire about the eating habits of the person being tested. When a patient's M-Field suggests sugar handling stress, the dialogue goes something like this: "The body seems concerned about your ability to handle sugar. Have you been getting a lot of sugar in your diet recently?" The answer to that question determines what the next question will be.

When exploring the source of the sugar handling stress, it can feel like playing the game of "20 Questions" with a patient. The goal is to determine whether the sugar handling problem is based around a recent isolated event, such as a birthday party, or whether it is just the *tip of the iceberg*. For many people, sugar is a much larger problem than an occasional indulgence. A 2009 article in Circulation magazine, published by the American Heart Association, revealed that the average intake of added sugars was as high as 34.5 teaspoons per day for some segments of the population. Their recommended limit is 6-9 teaspoons per day.

Sugar handling is one of the many health issues that require a two-step intervention. The first and most important step is to counsel the patient about the importance of recognizing and avoiding the sources of sugar in their diet. The next step is to identify nutritional supplement solutions that may help support the important sugar handling organs and glands. Some supplements, such as Inositol or Gymnema can even help the patient to control their sugar cravings. While nutritional or herbal support for the pancreas, liver and adrenal glands can be incredibly helpful in sugar handling, the long-term health of the patient depends upon whether or not they can get control of their sugar habits.

One of the diagnostic tools available in modern medicine is called a Positron Emission Tomography (PET) scan. In the management of cancer patients, PET scans are often used to locate cancerous tumors and monitor them. Radioactive glucose is used to track the progress of tumors because the sugar will immediately travel to the site of the tumor. As early as the 1930s, it was known that sugar is "food" for cancer. Although it has usually been recommended that cancer patients be given instructions to "watch their diets", according to the National Academy of Science, it is only recently that patients report being informed that sugar actually feeds cancer. If I was a cancer patient, I certainly would want to know this fact. As a natural healer, I share it with everyone, cancer patient or not.

Fortunately, the MFT protocols contain a large number of nutritional "tools" that assist the body in regulating blood sugar. The energy signatures of these supplements are found in the vials of the MFT Foundations Kit. In this way, we can easily identify any energetic issues and respond to them quickly and accurately with the proper supplementation and dietary guidance.

Avoiding Fructose and High Fructose Corn Syrup

Before we leave the subject of sugar handling, I would like to make one more appeal to anyone who will listen about avoiding fructose and especially high fructose corn syrup.

High fructose corn syrup (HFCS) is the number one source of calories in the United States. Although the industry that manufactures it is fond of claiming it is natural, it is actually a highly processed product that could never exist in nature. Much of the commercial HFCS is produced using a caustic soda *contaminated with mercury*. Detectable levels of mercury were found in over 30% of the commercial products that contained HFCS (Mercola).

Like many of the other artificially developed products, our MFT testing experience shows that high fructose corn syrup has an energy signature that is incompatible with the human body. HFCS creates an M-Field reaction similar to that of known poisons such as mercury and arsenic. We are unsure whether this is due to the processing, the mercury or some other contaminant. When I see this reaction from any substance, my advice will always be the same: DO YOUR BEST TO AVOID IT!

Avoidance is now very difficult in our society, since HFCS is included in most processed food products. Lately, the farmers who grow the corn, the big food conglomerates who process the corn, and even our own government have been "circling the wagons" with television and magazine marketing campaigns defending HFCS. *I think they know we're on to them.*

Despite the television commercials that claim that there is no difference between HFCS and cane sugar, the M-Field energy signature matching test demonstrates an obvious energetic difference. Now the HFCS lobby has started another campaign to change the name from "high fructose corn syrup" to "corn sugar". The public relations campaign by the purveyors of HFCS may want you to believe that the name is being changed so that people can make better dietary decisions. Whatever candy-coated-turnip truck they think we fell off of, it is plain to see this is far from the truth.

As consumers have become increasingly suspicious of HFCS, the manufacturers have turned up the heat on their marketing. "Corn sugar" has a wholesome, natural-sounding ring to it. It remains to be seen what levels they will stoop to in their attempts confuse the public, but we can be certain we have not heard the last of it.

Chapter 12

The Importance of Mineral Balance

"God sleeps in the minerals, awakens in plants, walks in animals, and thinks in man."

–Arthur Young

Vitamin deficiency is a well known problem, with various micronutrients taking center stage as new studies come out to isolate and examine their effects. Recently, vitamin D is getting a lot of press, appearing on health news segments and gracing the covers of popular magazines.

Less popular but equally important is the problem of mineral deficiency. The most talked about mineral is calcium, as it should be since there is far more calcium than any other mineral in the human body. Minerals have been subject to the same lack of differentiation and confusing marketing ploys that characterize American dietary trends, but to a lesser degree.

While thumbing through Reader's Digest, the reader comes across an article about the necessity of increasing the intake of dietary calcium to prevent osteoporosis. Motivated by what they've read, the reader then makes a trip to the drugstore and searches the aisles for a calcium supplement. Since Reader's Digest made no differentiation between organic calcium and inorganic calcium, the consumer is not particularly interested in the source of the calcium. The goal, after all, is just to buy some calcium and begin to take it.

A year goes by and it is time for their annual physical. The doctor decides to repeat the same bone density test in which this person scored so low last year. Of course, the patient is positive that the results this year will be much better because of their dedicated calcium supplementation. The results are in: The bone density score is worse than last year! How can this be when they have been taking all this calcium?

Sadly, I have heard this story many times over the years.

Organic Minerals vs. Inorganic Minerals

Mineral balance in the body is extremely important, and there are many factors involved in optimum mineral nutrition. The most important is the source of the minerals: the body can only utilize minerals that are organic, as opposed to minerals that are "inorganic".

An organic mineral is *a mineral that has been acted-upon by a living cell*, while an inorganic mineral is *a mineral that has **not** been acted-upon by a living cell*. In other words, it is just another rock, which cannot be processed by our bodies. As a plant grows out of the soil, it transforms the minerals from inorganic to organic, making them functional for humans.

Some of the confusion on the subject of minerals may be because of the way the word "organic" has been co-opted in contemporary language. *Organic* was originally a chemistry term used to describe a molecule that is carbon-based, meaning it contains a *carbon atom* in the molecule. All living things on the planet are carbon-based. Therefore, if it was ever *living* on planet earth, it can be called organic in the traditional sense of the word.

The word inorganic is also used in chemistry to describe a molecule that does not contain carbon atoms. That would indicate that it has never been associated with any living form, such as a plant or animal.

In modern verbiage, the word *organic* is used to describe food that was grown on soil without chemicals, herbicides or pesticides. 200 years ago, all food was "organic", but nobody used that term. A word to differentiate wholesome food from contaminated food was created out of necessity.

Although there are government rules dictating organic food labeling, there is no strict definition of the phrase *organic food*. In America, the United States Department of Agriculture (USDA) decides what food is *organic* and what is *not organic*. Some consumer groups, at odds with the USDA's definition and regulation of term "organic", have developed their own independent standards for organic certification. It is reasonable to assume that the USDA can be subject to the same lack of political integrity as the Food and Drug Administration (FDA). Once again, the issue comes down to trust. Under the current federal standards, consumers must be able to trust our government agencies in order to trust the label *organic*.

Depleted Soil makes Depleted Food

Labels aside, the problems with mineral deficiency run deep. The mineral content of our vegetables is now estimated to be approximately one-half of what it was just 50 years ago. This is due in part to the use of petroleum-based fertilizers which provide nitrogen to the soil but do not replenish depleted minerals. According to Purdue University Professor Dr. Don Huber, another factor is the herbicide *glyphosate*, which is the most commonly used herbicide in the US. Glyphosate *chelates* the minerals in the soil, changing their composition and leaving them unable to be absorbed by the vegetables. Given the prevalence of glyphosate in industrial applications, modern farming, and home gardening, combined with the long-term use of petroleum-based fertilizers, it is reasonable to assume that the average American is now chronically deficient in minerals.

Organic minerals, which are the only kind the body can efficiently put to use, must come from whole food. The best food sources for high mineral content include organic vegetables, mineral water, quality sea salt and bone broths. The mineral supplements for sale at the local drugstore are most likely inorganic, meaning they originated from rocks, not from food. In the MFT Foundations Test Kit, there are many energetic vials that represent organic whole food minerals. There is no point in testing for mineral deficiency using inorganic energies because the body has no use for them, therefore they will not match the energy signature of the M-Field.

Make No Bones about It! Minerals are Important!

There are seven macro-minerals in the body: calcium, phosphorus, potassium, magnesium, sulfur, sodium, and chloride. Minerals normally make-up about 4% of our total body mass. They are important for the strength of bones, with calcium at the forefront as ninety-nine percent of it is stored in the bones. The mineral composition of the bones also plays a role in pH balance, the acid-base equilibrium of the body. Specifically, the mineral chloride is an important factor in pH, as it is needed to make hydrochloric acid. Other minerals assist in nutrient transport across cell membranes, helping to feed the cells while still others help maintain osmotic pressure balance.

One of the most important physiological functions of minerals is the assistance provided in contraction and relaxation of the skeletal muscles. The same can be said for that most important muscle, the heart. Additionally, the minerals, especially calcium, are necessary for proper nerve conduction. Since the nervous system runs the body, mineral deficiencies can have serious consequences for homeostasis, the body's ongoing process of chemical balance.

Some interesting symptoms can come about as a result of a specific mineral deficiency, including leg cramps, heart palpitations, low thyroid, problems with temperature regulation, digestive distress, osteoporosis, swollen feet, insomnia, irritability, headaches, high blood pressure, fatigue, anemia, cold hands and feet, and muscle spasms, just to name a few.

How many times have you visited the medical doctor with one or more of these symptoms and been given medication for symptom relief? If your answer is one or more times, it would be wise to consider mineral deficiency as a potential cause of the symptoms. Consider it from the perspective of Dr. Weston Price's research. Unless your diet is considerably different from that of your neighbors, you are mineral deficient. The real question becomes, which mineral deficiency is causing which symptom?

The MFT Foundations Kit includes organic mineral energies to immediately assess the mineral needs of the body and to respond to those needs with organic minerals from a trusted source. The MFT method of addressing mineral balance has resulted in many happy stories about improvement in bone density tests and many other seemingly unrelated conditions.

Chapter 13

General Toxicity

"I love trash!"

~Oscar the Grouch

Any discussion of cellular health would not be complete without consideration of the toxins that can *inhibit normal cellular reproduction.* Even when the nutrients are present and plentiful, if there are contaminants in the body, cellular health will be compromised. The last section in the MFT Foundations Kit is named *Autotoxemia,* defined as *toxins that have been ingested or absorbed* which the body would like to eliminate. More appropriately, this section of the kit could have been called, "*Solutions* for Autotoxemia", because all of the energies in this section of the Foundation Kit represent common nutritional supplements known to rid the body of toxins. In natural health care, these are called "drainage remedies", and they are also commonly used in *detoxification* or *purification* treatments.

In order to build healthy cells, toxins need to be purged from the body. Our *cellular construction project* example likened it to building a new house at the city dump. There are many times when patients wish to become healthy by ingesting high quality nutrients, but that process is blocked by the toxic buildup from years of ingesting *poisons.* In our analogy, we must first clean up the construction site *or get rid of the toxins.* Then we can bring in our *raw materials,* also known as the nutrients, and plenty of sets of blueprints (the Protomorphogens™), to begin our soon-to-be-successful cellular construction project.

When the Autotoxemia Section of the Foundations Kit is the body's *priority,* as indicated by the *interested muscle response,* it is a good idea to begin the patient's nutritional protocol with a specific form of detox. Fortunately, the M-Field will tell us what the most efficient solution is through the use of the Morphogenic Field Technique. However, knowing what to do for the toxicity is only solving half the problem. Every toxic situation in the body requires two steps: helping the toxins drain out of the body with a drainage remedy, AND identifying the source of the poisoning or toxicity for the purpose of avoiding future exposure.

Drainage Remedies

Similar to *scar therapy*, drainage therapy is more popular in Europe than it is in the United States. Perhaps this is because of the **disease-oriented** approach of the American system of health care. In European countries such as Germany and Italy, where the emphasis is more on *health* as opposed to *illness*, it is much more common to use nutritional, herbal or homeopathic remedies that encourage the body to release built-up cellular toxins. They are generally safe and quite effective when recommended by skilled practitioners.

The superiority of the European health care system is no secret, even to our own military, which has often sent wounded soldiers there for rehabilitation. In war, soldiers can be exposed to a variety of chemicals and toxins in the combat zone, and of course, battle-wounds become battle-scars. The German medical system is known for its scar therapy and detoxification programs using drainage remedies to assist the body's *organs of elimination*.

The organs of elimination are those organs which help rid the body of the metabolic wastes which are byproducts of normal physiology. Examples include the liver, the kidneys, the lymphatics, the large intestine and the skin. When these organs are working efficiently, wastes are also eliminated from the body efficiently. When they are not working efficiently, the toxins can back up into the body and become static. A backup of toxins creates the *city dump effect* referred to in the cellular construction project analogy.

Mountains and Molehills

One of my greatest frustrations in dealing with American health care occurs when many of the easy, natural solutions that would create true health are ignored in favor of costly alternatives. All too often, the first line of defense is expensive, high tech diagnostic procedures that ultimately lead to expensive, high tech medical procedures, or drug protocols using patented pharmaceuticals that are later recalled because of serious side effects and adverse reactions. These interventions are frequently considered an acceptable gamble, while a safe medicinal herb is dismissed as "unproven."

We often read about some of the flaws in the medical system. A recent article in the New York Times online edition described a study authored by the Inspector General of the Department of Health and Human Services. The study stated that only about one in seven medical errors with hospital Medicare patients are reported, including some events that caused patients to die. The study estimated that more than 130,000 Medicare beneficiaries experienced one or more *adverse events* each month.

Some medical organizations have asserted that medical mistakes are responsible for at least 100,000 deaths in this country each year, while others estimate this number to be much higher. If this was happening within any other profession, that profession would soon cease to exist. As an alternative health professional, I have witnessed how political medicine *tries to make a mountain out of a molehill* when another profession is involved in unintended consequences. Yet, when the pharmaceutical and medical industries are involved, they *try to make a molehill out of a mountain.*

There was a recent outcry following a segment on The Dr. Oz Show. Dr. Oz mentioned the high level of arsenic found in apple juice, the result of spraying pesticides on the apple trees. He received much criticism from many of his medical colleagues, since the FDA had previously implied that the levels of arsenic in apple juice were acceptable. In the end, Dr. Oz was proven right when the FDA was forced to admit that the statements he had made on the air were indeed correct.

Most of us considered apple juice a healthful drink. And most of us, though possibly misguided, put our faith in the government agencies that are responsible for protecting us from dangerous food. It must have been somewhat embarrassing for the FDA to admit that they had allowed this level of arsenic in a fruit juice that is readily consumed by American children. To their credit, once the FDA was painted into a corner, they did admit that Dr. Oz was right. It was my privilege to witness an apology on the ABC Evening News from the network's medical consultant, who had previously been extremely critical of Dr. Oz for making this pronouncement.

Unfortunately, the apple juice is not an isolated case. The increase in pesticide and herbicide use in American agriculture is well documented. The FDA and the USDA isolate each vegetable or fruit toxicity as a separate event. But when considering the *collective accumulation of toxins* from all of the foods we consume that are grown in soil contaminated with pesticides and herbicides, it is frightening. Our FDA's policy toward allowable arsenic is totally unsustainable.

The frequency of autoimmune diseases has risen on parallel trajectories with the increased use of chemicals. We are all at risk. So how do you protect yourself?

This is the question addressed by the MFT Autotoxemia section. All of the drainage remedy supplements found in this area of the Foundations Test Kit support the body's need to purge chemicals and heavy metals. When these energies react during the MFT procedure, we consider this a request by the body to clean up the "toxic waste site" that is the result of living in our modern world.

For this reason, the last section in the Foundations Kit addresses the potential need for the body to detoxify through the use of drainage remedies. One of the most important nutritional supplements that work to eliminate toxins is Parotid PMG®. The parotid gland plays a role in the creation of saliva, which provides the enzyme amylase, essential for digesting complex carbohydrates. There is also a lesser known enzyme created in the parotid gland which has the ability to bind to metals and chemicals which are in the body and help escort them out.

The modern human body can be exposed to hundreds of chemicals in a single day. They are in every bite of food we eat, much of the air we breathe, and on many of the surfaces we touch. Therefore, the parotid gland needs all of the support it can get. Again, the MFT Procedure identifies the need *and* the solution.

In addition to Parotid PMG®, the test kit also includes the energy of Spanish black radish. I personally consider Spanish black radish to be the greatest single detoxification vegetable on the planet. High in sulfur, this unique radish has the ability to quickly and effectively reduce the toxic load in the lymphatics. Over the years, I have advised hundreds of patients to take Spanish black radish to counteract the symptomatic effects of refined and commercial food. When the patient has been on a junk food binge, it is not uncommon for them to have increased muscle aches, fatigue and headaches. Spanish black radish, along with avoidance of these foods, can result in an almost miraculous remission of symptoms within one or two days.

Recommending Spanish black radish is somewhat of a double-edged sword. It provides relief so fast and complete that the patient may not take the dietary exposure problem seriously, and consequently may not make the necessary changes to their lifestyle.

Another effective drainage remedy is fenugreek. Lymphatic toxicity, combined with cooler seasonal weather can create thick sludgy mucous. A buildup of mucous in the throat, sinuses, mastoid, lungs and intestinal tract can be quickly relieved by using fenugreek. Of course, we only recommend it when the energy signature of the fenugreek matches the energy signature of the person being tested. When the energies match, the person usually feels much better within a day or two.

Although short-term detoxification programs can provide a great deal of symptomatic relief, a prolonged program of methodical detoxification or purification is much more beneficial. Also contained in the Autotoxemia section of the test kit is a vial that represents the energy of the Standard Process® Purification Program. As a part of her nutritional therapy practice, Autumn conducts a periodic series of classes to take several of her clients through *group purification*.

This is a three week process and the results can be life changing. When her clients have finished with the program, it is a revelation for them to discover how great their body can feel and how much energy they can actually have. The average person loses 10 to 15 pounds. The weight loss aspect of purification can be credited with the role fat cells play in buffering the level of toxicity in the blood stream. In order to get toxins out of the blood, the body will store them in fat. The more toxic the diet and environment, the more fat is required to assist in circulatory buffering. Weight loss comes easily for a body with few toxins, since there is no need to hold on to unnecessary fat. It is good to be purified!

Chapter 14

The MFT Immune/Autotoxemia Kit

"What is the essence of America? Finding and maintaining that perfect, delicate balance between freedom 'to' and freedom 'from'."

~Marilyn vos Savant, in Parade

While some of the general solutions for toxicity have been briefly discussed, it is also important to become familiar with the veritable smorgasbord of toxins available to us. These topics can be uncomfortable to discuss; it will require the revelation of suppressed facts which some people would rather not know. However, this information is absolutely essential to motivate change and reverse what is happening to the food supply in our country.

For ease of use, the three test kits are color coded red, white and blue. They are tested in that order to match the body's customary priorities. After addressing the foundational needs of the cells and screening briefly for general toxicity with the Foundations (Red) Kit, the next step is to test using the cellular energies, called the Morphogenic Proteins (White) Kit, looking for specific cellular needs. The third and final kit of the MFT Basic Procedure is the MFT Immune/Autotoxemia (Blue) Kit, which focuses on identifying the specific *things your body **has** but does not **want***.

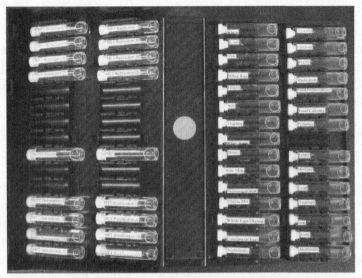

**The MFT Immune/Autotoxemia kit (the "Blue Kit") contains
the energies of cellular toxins and immune challenges.**

The health challenges addressed in the Immune/Autotoxemia test kit are
organized into two categories, with common immune problems on one
side, and environmental toxins on the other. The environmental toxins
are divided into three main areas: common food sensitivities, chemical
exposure, and heavy metal toxicity. Each of these areas represents an
epigenetic threat that has been rising steadily over the past century.

As the quality of food has degraded over the years, the body has taken
notice. Reactions to food are becoming increasingly common, with
symptoms such as skin rashes, sinus and migraine headaches, emotional
and behavioral problems, and countless others. The very thing that is
intended to nourish the body has instead become its enemy!

In addition to the poisonous food, the environment is another source
of toxins that wreak havoc in the body. We all absorb a wide range of
chemicals through the skin when we are exposed to cleaning solutions,
personal care products, and common household materials, such as carpet
and linoleum. In spite of its incredible ability to adapt, the body can no
longer handle the onslaught of chemicals from its current environment.

Heavy metals also creep in and cause a wide variety of symptoms, which
vary from person to person depending on the level of exposure and the

body's ability to buffer them. While trace amounts of some metals such as copper, zinc, and manganese are essential for wellbeing, metals such as lead and mercury are toxic. Stealth sources of heavy metals can be introduced through the use of silver/mercury amalgam dental fillings, inorganic mineral supplements, aluminum cookware, aluminum foil and aluminum chlorhydrate in anti-perspirants, to name a few.

And finally, there is a new recurring theme in the area of Autotoxemia; one that merits a chapter all its own. That theme is GMO's.

Mankind has developed the ability to take the food we have always known and turn it into something entirely different at the genetic level, a process known as "genetic engineering". The official policy of the U.S. Government since the inception of this technology is that *it should be pursued and developed for commercial purposes*. Along the way, there have been many scientists who have supported it, while many others have questioned the probable long-term consequences of this effort.

Since genetic modifications have occurred in the vast majority of commercial foods, it is important to understand the history of how all this came about. As individuals and as a country, we must recognize the perceived advantages and the real dangers to altering our food supply. The truth is that genetic changes are forever! *Forever is a longtime to live with an experiment that has never been regulated or controlled yet has the power to alter the lives of our children, our grandchildren and every generation thereafter.*

Daunn's Story

> *How did I become a patient of Boulevard Natural Wellness? Well, I will tell you. I had known Autumn Smith for many years and had heard about Dr. Springob from his many other patients, but I had never really taken the time to find out what their office was really about. This is the story about how I finally got a clue. I had been diagnosed with Premenstral Dysphoric Disorder (PMDD), Fibromyalgia, Clinical Insomnia, and most recently, Irritable Bowel Syndrome (IBS). I had spent countless hours and way too much money (no health insurance) on trying to deal with my "diagnoses". I just wanted to know what was really wrong with me. After*

another particularly frustrating doctors' appointment I was venting to Autumn that I'd had enough. The last doctor (of seven I might add) had just given me his thoughts on my situation. I had just told him of my symptom: three straight years of constant, severe nausea, morning and night. His pearl of wisdom was to ask me, "are you sure you're not pregnant?" REALLY? Apparently he'd missed the 3 year part. Autumn sat and listened patiently while I grumbled, and then offered her thoughts. "Why don't you come to our office and see if Dr. Frank can help you?" I thought, "Great…another person that just won't listen!" "I don't need my back popped honey, I feel like I'm gonna throw up!" She tried to explain to me that what they offered was way more than an adjustment, but I just didn't understand.

I went home that night even more frustrated than ever. I lay up all night (insomnia) and by morning I figured what did I have to lose? I gave every other "crackpot" a chance, why not just one more? So I called and made my appointment and gave it a skeptical try. My first visit was not at all what I expected and I honestly felt like it was complete non-sense. Using my energy field? Muscle testing? Aww Jeez! What had I gotten myself into? But I kept making them explain it until it started to make sense. I bought a bottle of Spanish Black Radish and within a week I was nausea free!!! After three YEARS! Turns out I had a "gummed up" gallbladder! That's it!!! Spanish Black Radish took care of the "I.B.S." Within a year of working monthly with Dr. Springob and weekly with Autumn I was sleeping through the night, discovered I did not have "Fibromyalgia", I was actually just allergic to genetically modified foods (GMOs). Later, I started taking supplements for the missing essential fatty acids I needed in order to balance my endocrine system and guess what… No more "PMDD". With all my new found energy I was able to free myself of 65 pounds of extra body fat and finally start living the life I always wanted. It's been close to four years since Boulevard Natural Wellness and their Morphogenic Field Technique changed my life, and I'm thankful every single day I gave it a chance. Thanks for reading my story!

Chapter 15

The Many Energetic Problems with Genetically Modified Foods

"There is nothing wrong with America that cannot be cured by what is right with America."

-William J. Clinton

The industry that creates genetically modified foods has made many political inroads to the government regulatory agencies that oversee them. 40 years ago, my father, a World War II veteran, would have argued to his death that the U.S. Government could not possibly be involved in anything as sordid as the story you are about to be told. The fact that my generation could question the integrity of a U.S. government agency was appalling to my father. His country was above reproach.

I, on the other hand, was a child of the 1960's. I questioned everything, and I'm still doing it today. I love America and her fundamental tenets of a government by the people, for the people, and liberty and justice for all. It is my belief and commitment to these principles that makes me decry the corruption and greed that has driven the development of genetically modified food. While superficially there may be merits to genetic engineering, the proof is in the energy response. Time after time, when testing GMO energies with results that are 100% consistent, I can come to no other conclusion but that genetically modified food is something to be feared. Indeed, we are on "The Nutritional Eve of Destruction!"

In clinical practice, using the MFT energy signature testing procedure, I have been alarmed at the number of health conditions that seem to be related to the consumption of genetically modified foods (GM/GMO). When creating the test kits, we researched all the modern food variables to identify potentially harmful health effects from an energy perspective. Just as we included the energy of unhealthy hydrogenated fat in our testing procedure, we also created virtual energies of many other synthetic and processed foods that have the potential of creating some of the greatest health risks.

Because of the massive amounts of sugar being consumed by the average American, the energy of refined carbohydrates was an obvious place to look for health problems. Therefore, the virtual energy of sucrose, also known as table sugar, is included in the Immune/Autotoxemia Test Kit for toxic foods. Almost as an afterthought, we included the energy of the *genetic modification process* to the "Common Foods" portion of the test kit. Things got very interesting after we took this step. The GMO energy vial reacted negatively on every person that we tested.

Recall that in MFT terminology, an **energy vial attraction** is a bad thing, since it means that the M-Field has an *energetic concern* with the contents of that vial. This was the phenomenon we witnessed. When testing a vial, the M-Field's attraction indicates either a deficiency or a toxicity; the attraction we observed with the **GMO energy vial** revealed that it had a toxic energy reaction for everyone tested.

The autonomic nervous system should not show an interest in any vial containing normal energy. The M-Field **will reject all energies** that it is not *interested in,* as indicated by a weakened test muscle. If the M-Field shows an interest, as indicated by a strong test muscle, it means that the autonomic nervous system has an *energetic issue* with the virtual energy being tested. In the MFT procedure, a rejection of the energy vial of GMOs would be a good thing, since that would signify no concern. We would be supportive of the GMO concept if the energy tested well and was **consistently rejected** by the body.

While there are mountains of evidence against genetically modified organisms, the battle for our food supply wages on. For us, it is quite simple. Had the M-Field rejected the genetically modified energy, it would not be included in this book. As the co-developer of MFT, if the M-Field is not concerned with an energy, then neither am I.

The results of thousands of energy signature tests with genetically modified foods are consistent: there is something about them that the body does not like or want. In fact, the reaction of the GMO energy to the M-Field was exactly the same reaction that we would receive if the body was tested with common poisons such as arsenic or mercury.

When we began the initial experiments with genetically modified energies, the GMO vial was non-specific. We did not know exactly what about the GMO process was provoking the body's negative reaction. Soon it became obvious that we needed to differentiate the stages of the genetic modification process to clarify the GMO problems. We wanted to know if it was possible that there was just one "bad step" in the **GMO creation process,** or if all the steps were problematic. We also investigated if all of the steps were bad for everyone, or was it possible that certain steps were bad for certain people?

We had to consider all the possible problems with the GMO process in order to isolate which of these components were responsible for the energetic reactions we found. As we researched the steps taken in creating genetic modifications, the first question in this discovery process was, "Why did Monsanto genetically modify the seeds in the first place?"

The answer to this question became evident the more we learned about GMO's.

We discovered that the genetic modification process was implemented for many and varied reasons. After decades of controlling weeds with chemical herbicides, the crop yields were being affected by the poisoned soil. Some seeds, such as soy, had been genetically modified to grow better on the poisoned soil. This led us to wonder, was the poisoned soil responsible for the energetic attraction of the GMO energies? Or, was the genetic alteration of the seeds creating a unique energy that simply did not match the energy signature of the body?

Another possibility was the genetic modification process itself. Could "the promoter" be responsible for the M-Field's reaction to the GMO energy vial? The promoter is the virus-based creation used to initiate the genetic changes needed to change the seed. Or possibly, it was a combination of all three factors (the herbicides, the genetically altered seeds and the promoter)? There is also the additional possibility that other unknown factors in the process were responsible for the M-Field reaction. We had a lot yet to consider.

To sort out this myriad of possibilities, we called again upon our virtual energy master, Dr. Nick Lamothe. Nick agreed to isolate all the known variables into individualized energy vials. In this way, we could test each of these energies individually to clarify which part of the GMO process was responsible for the energetic incompatibility that was evident on every person we had tested.

Upon receiving the individualized GMO vials, we placed them into prototype test kits. Over the next few weeks and months, we tested hundreds of people with combinations of GMO energies. One of our goals was to match the GMO "problems" with potential GMO "solutions".

What we discovered was that the reaction of the M-Field to the various components of the GMO process was a matter of the individuality of the person being tested. In keeping with the basic premise of MFT, the reactions and the responses both depended upon the biochemical individuality of the patient. There was not just one problem. There was not just one solution.

GMO Problem #1:
Poisoning the Soil for Fun and Profit

Most people who go to the grocery store in our modern age probably do not spend a lot of time pondering what may be hidden within the fresh vegetables. If they did, it would mean they were aware of the common practice of growing our commercial vegetables in glyphosate-contaminated soil. The more I learned about the herbicide glyphosate, also known as Roundup, the more suspicious I became in the produce department.

In modern organic farms, a great deal of human effort goes into making sure the weeds do not overrun the cash crop. An entry level job at the large organic whole food supplement company, Standard Process®, is that of "weed puller". On the Olympic Peninsula, organic farmer Nash Huber oversees many acres of organic fields. In order to control weeds on his farms, Nash uses the customary methods of pulling the weeds by hand or with a hoe. In addition, his crew burns them off with propane torches at an appropriate time just as the cultivated seeds are starting to sprout. He says that this give the new seeds about one week head-start on the weeds.

This practice is labor intensive to be sure. Done in order to maintain his organic certification and still control the weeds, these strategies are among the approved methods. Commercial farms are known for applying large amounts of herbicide onto the soil to control the weeds. Of course, this means that the plants grown on the soil will absorb some of the herbicide, especially root crops such as carrots and beets.

The most commonly used herbicide, Roundup, is produced by Monsanto. They also produce a genetically modified (GM or GMO) soy seed. The purpose of the genetic modification is to allow the soy plant to grow better on soil sprayed with Roundup. Though this may sound great in theory, there are multiple problems that result: it allows for the addition of even more herbicide to the soil, and it changes the genetic make-up, and therefore the energy, of the soy seed.

The MFT energy signature matching test demonstrates the energetic difference between organic soy and genetically modified soy. The difference in the muscle response to these two types of soy is dramatic. While most human bodies are accepting of the energy from the organic soy, the GMO soy response is the same as the response to the energy of arsenic.

Research science confirms the difference as well. Jeffery Smith, the director of the Institute for Responsible Technology, reports that a Brazilian study found that female rats fed GMO soy for 15 months showed significant changes in their uterus and reproductive cycles, compared to rats fed organic soy or those given no soy. According to United Kingdom senior pathologist Dr. Stanley Ewen, something in a GM soy diet was "wrecking" the ovary and endometrium of the rats. In his analysis of the data, Dr. Ewen strongly suggested one possible cause is the weed killer used on the GM soy beans.

This is just one of a number of studies done outside the United States that confirm that genetically modified soy and its counterpart glyphosate have significant impact on hormones in test animals. Although humans are not test animals, these findings have serious implications for the women who eat GMO soy. Further testing would be required to differentiate whether the hormonal problems were coming from the fact that the seeds have been genetically modified or from the fact that they were grown in soil poisoned with tremendous amounts of glyphosate. Monsanto, however, has a history of not allowing outside testing on their patented seed varieties.

Where there is GMO soy, there is glyphosate; they were literally made for each other! Monsanto's version of genetically modified soybeans is called "Roundup Ready". The seeds have a bacterial gene inserted which allows the plants to survive a normally deadly dose of Roundup Herbicide. And although this application does not kill the plant, the active ingredient, glyphosate, accumulates in the beans themselves which are then consumed by humans.

Jeffery Smith further states that there is so much glyphosate in GM soy beans that when they were first introduced to Europe, the regulatory agencies had to increase their allowable glyphosate residue levels by 200 fold. Although there are only a handful of studies on the safety of GM soy beans, there is considerable evidence that the poisoned soil wreaks havoc with the endocrine and reproductive systems.

When responding to a question about how glyphosate destroys plant life, Smith responded, "The herbicide doesn't destroy plants directly. It rather cooks up a unique 'perfect storm' of conditions that revs up disease-causing organisms in the soil, and at the same time wipes out plant defenses against those diseases. The mechanisms are well-documented but rarely cited."

Another problem that is rarely talked about is the effect on mineral content in the plants grown in soil containing glyphosate. One of the actions that make glyphosate an effective herbicide is that it deprives plants of certain minerals by chelating them. These minerals include iron, zinc, copper, manganese, magnesium, calcium, and boron.

As mentioned earlier in the discussion of the importance of proper mineral balance, the food grown in this soil can be deprived of useable forms of the minerals that are necessary for human health. By eating these mineral-deprived foods, we become mineral-deprived as well, leaving us vulnerable to a long list of disorders and diseases. According to Jeffrey Smith:

> Glyphosate-induced mineral deficiencies can easily go unidentified and untreated. Even when laboratory tests are done, they can sometimes detect adequate mineral levels, but miss the fact that *glyphosate has already rendered them unusable.* Glyphosate can tie-up minerals for years and years, essentially removing them from the pool of nutrients available for plants, animals, and humans. If we

combine the more than 135 million pounds of glyphosate-based herbicides applied in the U.S. in 2010 with the total application over the past 30 years, we may have already eliminated millions of pounds of nutrients from our food supply.

With all of the documented environmental damage done by the products of Monsanto, it is little wonder that they were named the "worst company in the world" in 2012 by Natural Society. This dubious distinction is granted for, "threatening both human health and the environment." Monsanto alone earned a whopping 51% of the vote, while the thousands of other companies in the world shared the other 49%.

When the energy of glyphosate is found to be an issue during the MFT testing procedure, the *energetic solution* to the *energetic problem* is usually Parotid PMG®. Nutritionally, Parotid PMG® is used to support the body's ability to purge undesirable chemicals and heavy metals. Once again, when solving health problems created by toxins, a two-pronged approach is required: the addition of the nutritional supplement that supports the body in eliminating the poison, and the avoidance of the toxin in any and all forms. In this case, that would call for the patient to avoid commercial vegetables which have been grown on soil with glyphosate. In the United States, that essentially means anything that is not declared to be organic.

GMO Problem #2:
Altering Genetics Changes Everything

Many of the problems related to glyphosate are just the tip of the iceberg. The research indicates that food that has been genetically modified has irreversible changes to its *atomic structure* compared to that of *heritage food*. One of the crops this is most apparent in is soy.

The ingredient labels on almost any packaged commercial food include soy. Current law does not force manufacturers to add the words "GMO Soy" to the label. Since approximately 93% of the soy grown in the U.S. is genetically engineered, if you eat processed food, you are eating this type of soy.

It has been revealed that much of the "protein quality" information regarding GMO soy is unknown. Scientists are prohibited from evaluating the protein contained in the GM version of soy because Monsanto holds the patent on the seed. If testing was allowed outside of their laboratories, the resulting truth about the nature of the protein in the soy would make this story even more alarming. As it turns out, before testing was stopped, it was learned that the protein composition of genetically modified soy was unlike anything seen in nature.

After World War II, soy became a more common crop grown in United States, partly due to the high level of protein it was known to contain. Even with all of the modern health problems relating to commercial soy, there is one argument that can be made in favor of organic soy: it has some of the highest protein-content of any plant. From this perspective, it is valuable; for the vegetarian, life without high protein soy becomes difficult.

Nobody argues about the *quantity* of protein found in soy. With GM soy, the discussion becomes about the *quality* of the protein. One of the biggest concerns of people with food allergies is sensitivity to normal protein from natural grain sources. What can happen to these same people when the grain protein is a man-made creation instead?

In the 1990's, when GMO soy was first introduced in England, there was an immediate 50% increase in allergies to soy. Why? As it turns out, when seeds are genetically modified, their protein make-up is altered because amino acid chains cannot be controlled. This molecular manipulation resulted in the creation of protein molecules that have never been witnessed before. Since the human body had never been exposed to genetically engineered protein, great new risks of allergic-type reactions emerged.

The clinical results of the MFT Testing Procedure indicate that allergic-type reactions to GMO soy are commonplace. In our experience, it is one of the top-three food sensitivities, along with glyphosate and GMO corn.

There are many other GMO problems which must be addressed. Beyond soy, there are significant issues with GMO corn. Most people consume much more corn than they realize. Corn is prevalent. It is in the obvious places such as chips and breakfast cereals, but it is also in almost every soda, condiment, bread, granola bar, cracker, and juice on the market. Even if you avoid these snack foods, corn creeps in to the meat, egg, and dairy aisle. As the primary ingredient in the diet of industrially farmed animals, when we eat a steak from a corn-fed cow, or the eggs from a corn-fed chicken, we are eating corn. Like it or not, almost all of us are regularly consuming great amounts of food product that originated as GMO corn.

Approximately 85% of the corn grown in United States has been genetically engineered either to survive an application of herbicide or to produce an insecticide called Bt (short for Bacillus thuringienses). In other words, GM corn is genetically engineered to produce a toxin. Unless the corn or corn products you consume are certified organic by the USDA, nearly all of the food you buy will contain either GMO corn or soy or both, as is the case with most crackers and chips, which list both high fructose corn syrup and soy lecithin in the ingredients.

Recently, a group of Canadian researchers tested pregnant women for the presence of the Bt pesticide that is produced by GM corn. A doctor at Sherbrooke University Hospital in Quebec found the Bt-toxin in the blood of 93% of the pregnant women studied. It was also found in 80% of the umbilical blood in their babies. This peer reviewed study was published in the medical journal "Reproductive Toxicology" in 2011 (Mercola).

How tragic that these babies have been denied their God-given right to start life with a new "pure" body. Essentially, because of this previously unknown factor in the food their mothers consumed, these babies will be born with an abnormal and unnecessary toxic load.

The companies who hold the patents to these "Frankenfoods" built them in a laboratory using genes from viruses and bacteria. They then manipulated the policies, thrust their perverted product onto an unsuspecting public with the permission of the government, and will not allow them to be tested for safety. The fact that these foods remain unregulated is an outrage! Yet Monsanto and other companies that genetically modified the seed simply hire spokespeople and lobbyists to explain why people should not jump to conclusions about these findings. For me, it was not a great leap, but a hard shove from behind as the facts have accumulated into a mountain of frightening evidence.

Although the GMO industry would like us all to believe that genetic engineering is a very exact and precise science, nothing could be further from the truth. The process works something like this:

The scientists, for example, decide that they want to create a corn plant that would produce its own pesticide. The assumed advantage is that the corn plant would be protected from the insects that could attack the plant. They take a gene from a bacterial or viral species and splice it into another species, hoping that the **new creation** would take on the desired effect. (Smith)

There are a lot of assumptions in this process. The genetic engineers assume that the new seed will do what it is designed to do. They also assume that the only consequence to this action is the intended one. Then they assume that they can and will obtain a patent for this new creation and control it in the future. *In their perfect world*, these assumptions would be correct, but we already know that this has not been the case.

To genetically engineer the corn, the creators utilized the genes of soil bacterium called Bacillus thuringiensis (Bt). Then the engineers altered it to increase its level of toxicity. Millions of copies of the gene were made and then combined with a piece of a virus (called the "promoter"). It is the "on" switch to activate the gene from that point on, 24/7, around the clock.

The next step is to take the millions of copies, put them (literally) into a gun and shoot them into a plate of millions of cells. Their hope is that some of the genes get into the DNA of some of the cells. Those cells are then cloned and used to grow plants. During this process, there is massive collateral damage to the DNA that creates even higher levels of toxins. (Smith) This may explain the Canadian study, where such high levels of Bt toxin were found in the pregnant women and their babies.

GMO Problem #3: Other Unintended Consequences

There has never been a clinical study done to determine the long-term effects of humans eating genetically modified foods. Neither has there been published post-market surveillance on the possible health effects from their long-term use. According to Jeffrey Smith, director of the Institute for Responsible Technology, there was one study done in the UK. Curiously, once all the data was collected, the study suddenly vanished. The results were never disclosed to the public.

It seems as if the countries who were the greatest supporters of these biotech food experiments, such as the U.S and the U.K., now feel they need to hide the facts about the negative effects of GMOs from the public. I believe the time is coming soon when all of this suppressed information will be released in a sudden burst, much like it was with the tobacco industry. But before this can happen, the regulatory agencies of these governments must be forced to look within and find the integrity to rise above their own embarrassment. Then, all the facts can be brought to light about what they have allowed.

Some may remember back in the 1980's when the amino acid supplement, L-tryptophan, was suddenly removed from the market. At the time, the FDA blamed a contaminated source from Asia for the deaths of over 100 Americans. According to an interview with Jeffery Smith in the South African investigative magazine, "Noseweek", a thorough inquiry of the origin of the contaminated L-tryptophan revealed that it <u>was created with genetic modification</u>.

In addition to the 100 people that died, another 5000 to 10,000 experienced sicknesses or disability caused by the genetically engineered L-tryptophan. According to this article, the FDA withheld this information from Congress and the public in an apparent attempt to protect the biotech industry.

In my professional practice in those days, I recommended L-tryptophan for certain patients who were having trouble sleeping. Whenever I made this recommendation to the appropriate person, the results had always been stellar. It had a calming effect on the nervous system and allowed people to get a restful night's sleep. As you may know, L-tryptophan is the amino acid responsible for people falling asleep after big Thanksgiving Day turkey dinner.

I had always wondered how something that worked so well in my clinical practice could suddenly be so "evil" as to merit its permanent removal from the shelves at the health food store. At that time, this seemed to be a heavy handed and totally uncalled-for action by the FDA. Now, having read this report from Jeffery Smith, it all makes perfect sense to me.

The FDA was not protecting us from an evil amino acid supplement; it was protecting itself from the embarrassment of having to explain how a product created by a process that they were endorsing could have these devastating consequences on so many people. With the motivation of the FDA becoming clear and the precedent set for genetically modifications gone awry, evaluating the effects of the GM process became our priority as we developed the MFT Test Procedure.

Therefore, the Morphogenic Field Technique Test Kit includes the energy of **the promoter**, the virus that **initiates the genetic cascade** during the genetic modification process. Some of our research indicated that **the promoter does not become inert** once it is introduced to the genetically modified food. It turns the switch "on" and it stays on, raising the possibility of **potentially dangerous unintended genetic consequences**.

If this was true, we reasoned, it would be possible for the promoter to continue creating genetic changes in the human body after a GMO food was consumed. Indeed, one small study was done which demonstrated that the intestinal flora was genetically altered when the promoter was introduced to a living system (Smith). As we began testing individuals using the *promoter energy vial*, we found that this seemed to be true in some of the people we tested. When the promoter reacts in combination with the energies of *bacteria, viruses, parasites, molds, yeasts and fungus* during the energy signature matching test, we conclude that this relationship is evidence of microbe energies that did not exist prior to the genetic modification. The energy of these new, previously unacknowledged "life forms" suggests that the body has no acquired immunity against these microbes. The health challenge created by this situation could have potentially devastating consequences for us all.

When these patients were informed of the findings, we included recommendations about avoiding genetically modified foods. We also recommended pre-biotics, pro-biotics and digestive enzymes for nutritional support. Universally, when these recommendations were followed, the patient's symptoms dramatically improved.

When teaching MFT Seminars to health care professionals, I like to tell the story of a particular patient with a problem related to the energy of the GMO promoter. Julie, who lives approximately three hours away from my office, made the long drive to get treatment for excruciating back and rib cage pain. She had been a patient for several years and had recently been through liver transplant surgery.

Julie had been put on the transplant list because of severe cirrhosis of the liver, although her doctors were at a loss to explain the origin of the cirrhosis. This otherwise healthy middle aged woman did not drink alcohol and had no history of drug abuse or hepatitis. In fact, her Mormon background precluded her from engaging in many of the activities that one might associate with a cirrhotic liver.

Shortly after her surgery, she began having severe episodes of lower back, flank and mid-back muscle spasms, with the pain radiating around the rib cage on both sides. When the pain first started, she went to a local chiropractor close to her home. She reported that the pain was so great, she could not handle the chiropractic treatments. Out of desperation, Julie was willing to make the long painful drive to our office searching for some relief.

It was immediately apparent that this was not entirely in mechanical problem with her spine. The pain and the spasms could not be isolated to a single irritated nerve, but were spread around a rather large area in the low to mid-back. On a pain scale of 0 to 10, Julie was at 9 or 10.

20 years ago, I would have taken one look at Julie and sent her back home not knowing what to do for her. But with the MFT energy signature testing protocol, we tested Julie and found the energy of a *genetically modified parasite* located in both her pancreas cells and her kidney cells. With these findings, it seemed apparent that Julie was suffering from referred pain from those organs, which created a reflex spasm in the spinal muscles.

This insight guided the treatment, but there was still one glaring problem. Having just received a liver transplant, Julie was taking medication to suppress the immune system so that her body would not reject her new liver. The question arose: could it be that a genetically modified parasite had attacked the liver? Furthermore, could it be that a related organism, now with assistance from the immune suppressing medication, was attacking her pancreas and her kidneys? There was no way to know for certain, but the energy was clear.

Although we had many natural tools to assist the body attempting to rid itself of parasites, I wondered if our attempts to handle these parasite energies might jeopardize her new liver. Nutritional supplements and herbs that are anti-parasitic would also boost immune function at a time when the medical profession was trying to suppress the immune system.

The other issue was that Julie lived far away from where I practiced. I would not be able to keep a close eye on her from that distance. Of course, her surgeon would probably not be impressed with what I considered to be my *brilliant deduction* about the cause of Julie's pain. And almost certainly, he would not be impressed with my assumption about the etiology of Julie's cirrhosis.

So Julie and I had a long talk. I told her I would try to help her, but I needed her to be committed to the plan of action that I was proposing. If she was <u>not</u> committed to it, she would need to seek help in a different way. Julie and her husband both agreed that we would start a trial using nutritional supplements that were known to be anti-parasitic and that also matched the energy signature that her body was emanating.

Within a few days, the back spasm was beginning to subside. On her next visit, I was able to give her the chiropractic adjustment in addition to performing the Morphogenic Field Technique protocol. On that date, we slightly altered the dose of anti-parasitic nutrition based upon how her immune system was handling the nutrition in conjunction with the anti-rejection medication she was taking.

This was not easy for any of us. To me, it was like walking a tightrope; helping the body to destroy the parasite energy without affecting her new liver. For Julie and her husband, John, it required a huge commitment to drive 300 miles a week to give this a chance to work. But in the end, the results were nothing short of miraculous. Now, two years later, Julie still looks and feels wonderful.

This story illustrates two important concepts. The first is the effectiveness of Morphogenic Field Technique and the M-Field Energy Signature Matching. The second is the frightening reality that the GMO promoter probably has the ability to genetically modify living cells inside the human body.

The question I constantly ask myself when these unique energies present in a patient during the MFT Testing Procedure is, "What would become of this person if we did not have the ability to identify these energy signatures in their bodies?"

Then, there's the follow-up question: "What if we did not have the nutritional supplement resources to reverse the damage being inflicted upon the public by GMO foods?" The answers are both humbling and enraging.

My conviction that people have the right to know about these potential dangers hidden within the food they consume each day gives rise to the final, most compelling question: "What about everybody else who does not have access to either the energy signature testing or the nutritional solutions to these problems?"

There are legions of people out there who have no idea that the Innate Intelligence of their body's M-Field is ready and willing to share information about the origin of their health issue. The energy signature testing, Morphogenic Field Technique, is a true quantum conversation with the cells of the body. It is as easy as *asking the body what it wants and then giving it what it asks for*. It sounds too simple, but as the indigenous people of the Olympic Peninsula and the many other non-Industrialized cultures have demonstrated throughout history, sometimes the simple answer is the best answer.

More than ever, our country needs to hear the truth about real food. Only organic whole food and organic whole food supplements can turn around the health care crisis in which we find ourselves. As our food, the key to our continued existence, is being destroyed right before our very eyes, only *we the people* have the power to put a stop to this! Thankfully, despite the grim scenario of the many problems with GM foods, there are viable solutions and a reason for hope.

GMO Solutions

Finally, the good news about genetically modified food! Once the public understands the dangers of consuming foods that were never meant to enter the human body, the free market system will eliminate them from the store shelves.

These foods have crept up on us for the last two decades. Currently, there are more than 30,000 food items that contain GM Soy, yet the public remains unaware. Like many other dangerous food products that have preceded GMOs, once the secrets are out, consumer buying habits start to change. Hydrogenated/trans fats are a good example for comparison. It took several decades for the public to realize that man-made fats were unhealthy, but once the health risks were uncovered, many consumers started to eliminate hydrogenated fat from their diet.

Deceptive marketing and manipulated research data continue to be a primary tool to confuse the public into buying things that harm us. However, consumers are becoming savvier all the time. Because of their track record of deceit, consumer groups have sprung up to create an opposing voice for every marketing campaign that lacks integrity. For example, watchdog groups have spent years looking at the commercials for children's sugary breakfast cereals and snacks.

This is also the case with GMOs. Although many anti-GMO groups are now springing up around the country, Jeffrey Smith's Institute for Responsible Technology has been at the forefront of this battle. Mr. Smith has authored two best-selling books on the subject of GMOs. I have used his material extensively in creating the anti-GMO segment of our professional seminars teaching Morphogenic Field Technique. Each time I have contacted the Institute for Responsible Technology for assistance, they have been eager to assist me every step of the way.

In 2011, I had the chance to attend Jeffery Smith's anti-GMO Speakers Training Workshop in Seattle. At the end of the class, I was allowed to demonstrate our energy signature matching technique to the class. Those that attended witnessed a modified muscle response test that demonstrated that the M-Field was perfectly happy with the energy signature of organic soy and corn. It was then contrasted with a follow-up demonstration of how incredibly unhappy the M-Field is with the energy signature of genetically modified soy and corn.

Smith believes that if we can get 5% of the American public to reject food that contains GMOs, we will have reached the "tipping point". He believes that farmers will refuse to grow genetically modified seeds and the commercial food manufacturers will see the error in their ways and start purchasing commodities that are not genetically modified. Only time will tell if this is true. In the end, I believe that genetically modified foods will become known for what they are.

As with any new science, there are stages of development. There is a delay between its development and the public knowledge of its existence. Then there is additional lag time between the public knowing it exists and judging its value. The final step come when the public knows that a product is dangerous and awaits the politician to respond to the will of the people.

Right now, the public knows the GMOs exist but some of them have not decided whether they are good or bad. Surveys indicate, however, that the public states overwhelmingly that they would not buy genetically modified food if they knew that it was genetically modified. They just don't know that most of the commercial products they are buying every day in the grocery stores are genetically modified. The FDA and the USDA do not require them to be labeled. For the consumer who wishes to avoid GMOs there are two alternatives; eat only USDA organic food, which is not supposed to have genetically modified ingredients or buy foods that are labeled "non GMO".

It is a bizarre situation we find ourselves in, where those who have tampered with the very atomic structure of our food make no disclosures, and the food that has been consumed by humans for millennia is forced to wear the out-of-the-ordinary label. As if the word *organic* described some kind of boutique-food that is only for elite grocery snobs and counter-culture hippies, traditional food has become the alternative, while the corporate product masquerades as the norm.

In Washington State, a bill to require the labeling of genetically modified food was introduced in 2012. In spite of the fact that the introduction of this bill was a surprise to the anti-GMO groups, a very effective grass-roots response was put together quickly. There was a great deal of national and international coverage by the media. Unfortunately, the bills died in both committees where they were introduced. According to the "GMO-Free Washington" website, the chairmen of both the State House and State Senate committees had received political contributions from Monsanto.

Labeling would be the beginning of the end for GMO's in Washington State and Monsanto is aware. Norman Braksick, president of Asgrow Seed Co., a subsidiary of Monsanto, was quoted in the Kansas City Star as saying "If you put a label on genetically engineered food, you might as well put a skull and crossbones on it." Other states have taken notice as well. At press time, California has a voter's initiative on the ballot and both Michigan and Vermont have anti-GMO legislation pending.

The most important step you can take as a consumer is to write your representatives in the federal government at all levels and demand that they assume their oversight role to initiate changes in the FDA and the USDA. While you're at it, demand Congressional Hearings to investigate how we got into this situation in the first place. The absence of oversight, political favoritism and a general lack of administrative integrity within these regulatory bodies is intolerable. The public has a right to know what they are eating. The time has come for us to stop being the guinea pigs and take back control of our food.

Again, I would like to thank the Institute for Responsible Technology for providing much of the information used to create this section of the book. For more information about what you can do to protect yourself and your family from GMO food, go to www.responibletechnology.org. They have many free downloads that can give you more information than I can possibly provide in this space. They have all of the facts to back it up.

My greatest hope is that you will be motivated in some way to join this crusade. It is my firm belief that turning this situation around is essential for our very survival. The continued spread of genetic engineering for profit has brought us to "the nutritional eve of destruction".

Kathy's Story

> In the winter of 2010, I was diagnosed with multiple sclerosis. I was 43 years old at the time of my diagnosis and my world came crashing down. Between the time of my diagnosis and the months that followed, I was not feeling better. I had to cut back on my work schedule. I was seeing another chiropractor at that time and he could not adjust me correctly because of the problem. I was a mess! My son recommended Dr. Springob and told me about his technique. He even made the appointment for me. He really felt Dr. Springob could help me.

> When I went in for my first appointment, one of the initial steps was to measure my energy level. I had absolutely no energy field at all. Because of my diagnoses, he tested me for heavy metals in my nervous system and spinal cord and

found that I had high levels of mercury in my system. He recommended that I have my mercury fillings removed and started me on some supplements that would help remove the mercury from my system.

After taking the recommended supplements and having my mercury removed, within a few months I was feeling so much better. My adjustments were working again and my nervous system was much happier. I continued to see Dr. Springob on a regular basis and he would continue to test my energy field.

He always seems to know what is going on with my body using his testing technique. I never have to tell him what is going on because he can tell me just by testing me. Just the other day when I saw him I wasn't feeling very well. He knew that, tested me, and discovered that "genetically modified soy" showed up as the reason for the small energy field. As it turned out, I had just had some soy that day in a coffee drink. He didn't know that until he tested me. He recommended a supplement and by the next day I was feeling much better. It is really amazing how this technique works---and it does work! I am a firm believer in MFT.

Since I started seeing him two years ago I've gone from part-time work back to full time. My energy level is high most of the time and I don't get that horrible fatigue that seems to plague most people with multiple sclerosis. I have hope now and feel that my disease can now be controlled through energy field testing. This type of health care has become a very important part of my recovery. I feel like I have my life back and I can now plan a future full of great possibilities.

Chapter 16

Sources of Autotoxemia #1: Common Processed Foods

"All our progress is an unfolding, like a vegetable bud. You have first an instinct, then an opinion, then a knowledge as the plant has root, bud, and fruit. Trust the instinct to the end, though you can render no reason."

~Ralph Waldo Emerson

The Morphogenic Field Technique blossomed from the right question asked at the right time. As it evolved, at times it seemed to take on a life of its own. The technique has changed my practice, as well as the practice of many professionals who have learned it. Most importantly, it has changed the life of patients. As with any life changing event, to make the most of the experience we occasionally have to go back and ask ourselves, "How did we get here?"

We got here primarily because as natural health practitioners, each day we encounter the effects of the toxic nature of many of the items that are making their way into our patient's bodies. MFT has evolved out of concern for the tremendous challenge we all face in keeping ourselves healthy in this modern world. As we developed the technique, Autumn and I aimed to fashion the optimum environment for regeneration of 60 billion cells each day. Cells make up the tissues, which make up the organs, which make up the organ systems of the *human organism*. As natural healers, we looked for the fastest, easiest and most accurate way of giving patients everything they needed to heal.

Autumn proposed a concept that was revolutionary in creating a new paradigm of healing. Instead of blood tests, instead of X-rays and MRI's or any of the other myriad of diagnostic tests and procedures, she proposed a conversation with the cells of the body from an energetic perspective. The purpose of the *quantum conversation* was to answer two important questions: What nutrients did the body need that it did not have? And what toxins did the body have that it did not want?

Further, in order to quantify the patient's progress over time, it was necessary to develop an *objective finding to* demonstrate to both the patient and the practitioner that the MFT process was having the intended effect. The "size" and "symmetry" of the human torus energy field, the M-Field, became our objective finding. The goal was growth of the diameter of the baseline M-Field from all directions. This measurement was accomplished by using a modified muscle response test and a supplement designed for the opposite gender.

The next step was to develop the *tools* needed to accomplish this task. We first developed the Morphogenic Protein Test Kit, which contains the virtual energies of 190 different types of cells. By combining these energies into 58 separate vials that represented an all-encompassing snapshot of the cells of the human body, we could then isolate the ones with *special needs.*

In addition, we created two M-Field Enhancement Vials to *ramp-up* the energy of the M-Field. One or the other of these vials created an *artificial increase* in the size of the M-Field. The increased size gave us increased information.

Our second test kit, the Foundations Test Kit, accomplished the goal of identifying foundational deficiencies of the nutrients that all cells require to grow and reproduce. The energies in this test kit address the body's needs in the areas of hydration, digestion, scarring, fatty acids, energy/sugar handling, minerals and the general concept of underlying toxicity that might prevent the body from fulfilling this process.

Toxicity can include challenges from exposure to genetically modified food, for example, but there may be other things *the body has picked up that it does not want,* a concept called "Immune/Autotoxemia."

The Immune/Autotoxemia Test Kit can be broken down into two main categories, which are separated into two sides of the test kit: *immune challenges*, which are the energy of the different microbes that can impact the body, and *toxins*, which are the poisonous energies found in the form of commonly consumed foods, chemicals, and heavy metals.

The individual categories of possible toxic foods found in the common Americans diet begin with the grains. Factors to consider are the biochemical individuality of the patient, as well as the quality and quantity of the grain being consumed.

Wheat Sensitivity

During the testing procedure, it is common for the M-Field to communicate distress regarding the offensive nature of grain energies. Wheat is the most common grain found in the American diet, the primary ingredient in the products that most people eat every day. These products include bread, breakfast cereal, pasta and crackers.

If the patient is given instructions to avoid wheat based upon an *M-Field Signature-Matching* test, the MFT practitioner must also be prepared for the long, sometimes difficult, discussion that will follow. Most people do not want to stop eating bread or bread products. A typical day for most of us includes toast with breakfast, a sandwich for lunch, crackers with soups, and rolls with their dinner. Therefore, when wheat turns out to be the offending food, life suddenly becomes a lot more difficult.

So what is it about the wheat that creates nutritional problems in the body from an *energetic perspective*? It may be the *gluten*, the protein component of the grain and the source of allergic-type sensitivity in many people. When informed about the energetic reaction to wheat, most people are not surprised, and often will acknowledge that eating wheat makes them feel bloated.

Considering the ongoing poisoning of the soil on American farms, I suspect that the herbicides and pesticides absorbed into the grains may be a factor in the reaction to the wheat. Another consideration may be the way the grain is handled. Often, it is stored in silos for long periods of time, and it may be sprayed with mercury to prevent fungus growth.

Prior to approximately 10,000 years ago, grains were not cultivated for human consumption. Just as our friends in Happy Valley 14,000 years ago consumed mostly animal fat, protein and "organic vegetables", there is an *evolutionary question* of whether grains should play a large role in the human diet. Is it possible that our digestive system was never adequately designed for processing grain?

Consider that grains are, in reality, the seeds of next year's wheat, rye or corn plant. In other words, when we eat grains, we are really eating seeds. How many seeds should one consume as part of their regular diet? As with all foods, it becomes an issue of moderation. Seeds (grains) in moderation may be healthy, but an excessive amount may create a physiological stress on the digestive system. Currently, the typical American diet contains more than a moderate amount of grain, especially wheat, and now GMO corn and soy.

The same seeds that offer nutritional benefits in moderation are habitually stripped of their assets before they make it into our food. Even organic wheat flour is simply what is left over after the nutritious bran and germ have been removed. Conversely, consider what happens when a seed is sprouted. No longer seeds, they have been transformed into nutrient-dense vegetables which are known to be easily digested. It takes a mere three days for wheat berries to become baby wheat plants, which can be baked into bread, pureed into smoothies, or just eaten raw.

To patients who test for wheat sensitivity during the MFT Procedure, I usually make the following suggestions: If you must have wheat, make sure it is organically grown to avoid the pesticides and herbicides which may be affecting it. Limit your consumption to just a few portions per week. Symptomatic improvement will be in proportion to your decrease in consumption; the less you eat, the better you feel.

GMO Corn and Soy

Although wheat is a common offender, without a doubt, GMO corn and soy are the most common foods that *create a reaction in* the M-Field. Occasionally, when either of these two grain energies react, the patient will ask whether or not the organic version of the grain would give the same result. This is an excellent question. To answer it, I keep samples of organic soy and genetically modified soy in my office so I can test each one separately on the inquisitive patient. I do not **tell them the difference**; I **show them the difference**.

Typically, the energy signature of the organic soy is compatible with the M-Field Signature-Matching test, but the GMO soy is not. The same is true for corn. Eighty-six percent of the corn in the American diet is genetically modified (Smith). Currently, although white corn is not yet genetically modified, unless it is organic, it is probably grown in soil containing pesticides and herbicides.

To clarify, GMO refers to the *seed* and organic refers to the *soil*. Since GMO seeds were developed to grow on poisoned soil, it makes no sense to grow GMO seeds on organic soil. The question we must ask ourselves as we shop for healthy foods is: if the seed is not genetically modified, is it still grown on poisoned soil? Most of the commercial grains and vegetables available in the grocery store have been grown on soils that are contaminated with pesticides and herbicides.

When these energies show themselves during an MFT test, my advice is a two-pronged approach of *avoidance of the offending food* combined with *taking the proper nutritional supplement* to help the body handle these adverse energies. Often the proper nutritional support requires both *drainage* of built-up toxicity along with an enzyme combination to *clean up the debris* left behind in the intestinal tract.

White Trash

Pejorative slang aside, I originally heard the term "white trash" in a lecture by Dr. Michael Dobbins in the 1990's. He used the term to describe the combination of refined white sugar, flour and rice. After noting that almost the entire population of America was consuming all of these on a daily basis, he explained the many reasons for limiting them in the diet. While I don't believe a lot of detail is required on this subject, I will make a recommendation that we all avoid eating them. In case it is not already obvious, these products are not real food, but a creation of man.

Honey

I like honey. Not in the same scale as Winnie the Pooh, but I have a little bit of honey three to four times a week. It is my one sweet indulgence. Although it does not often "test" as a problem, it is contained in our test kit. It is well known that it should not be given to infants because of the risk of botulism spores that can be present in honey.

My personal source of honey comes from the hives tended by my old friend and chiropractic school roommate, Dr. Meed West. Meed is an avid beekeeper and he is kind enough to supply my family with raw, unprocessed honey each year, even in the lean years of the honey harvest.

According to Meed, my trusted information source *for all-things-honey-related,* most honey that is purchased in the grocery store has been processed. Processed honey is often chemically refined, blended, and heated, which eliminates many of the beneficial vitamins and minerals. It is usually pasteurized, destroying the natural enzymes. If honey does not crystallize over time, it means that it has been heated to a high temperature that destroys nutrients. Additionally, commercial bee farms give their hives large doses of antibiotics to fight off disease. The residual by-products of these drugs are found in the honey. These factors may be responsible for the poor response that some people have to the energy of commercial honey.

It is quite difficult to get truly "organic" honey, because even under the best of circumstances, beekeepers cannot control where their bees forage. In these days of unbridled application of Roundup and chemical fertilizers, it is almost impossible to guarantee that bees have not been exposed to these toxins. However, unprocessed, raw, locally produced honey is a better option than most of the honey available in supermarkets.

Milk and Cheese

200 years ago, milk was radically different from what is purchased in the grocery store today. When describing dairy products, it is important to be very specific about which items within this category we are referring to. As nature intended, milk came from either a cow or goat that lived in an open area and grazed on what nature provided. The milk was extracted from the animal and consumed in varying forms, such as cheese, cottage cheese, cream or buttermilk.

Throughout time, this was the way it was until pasteurization, homogenization, "hormonization" (the act of feeding growth hormone to the cattle for the purpose if increased milk production) and other new concepts were introduced to the field of dairy farming. The same thing can be said about cheese, to an even greater degree. When it comes to purchasing dairy products these days, a good rule is *Caveat Emptor*: *Let the buyer beware*. Not only do most people have little idea about what they are purchasing, the differences between real milk and cheese and these processed products that once resembled milk are tremendous. Dairy products that are bought in most grocery stores are radically different from the milk and cheese that humans have consumed throughout history.

Similar to most other foods over the last 150 years, the commercial food industry has significantly altered our dairy products. To begin, the term "raw milk" can mean two radically different things. There is the **commercial** *raw milk* produced for the grocery stores, and then there is the **traditional** *raw milk* produced from organically raised, grass-fed cows. A vast difference exists between these two, yet both are called by the same name. The milk in your store comes from "conventionally raised" (but not traditional) grain fed livestock. What many people don't know is that cows were never meant to eat grain, they were meant to eat grass.

Cows that eat grain have problems that grass-fed cattle do not. Grain-fed cows are frequently given antibiotics to deal with the digestive problems created by the grain. Of course, this changes the nature (and the energy) of the milk. Additionally, these cattle are routinely given growth hormone to increase milk production, once again changing the nature of the milk. Unfortunately, there are only six states that currently allow the sale of organic raw milk and raw milk products. Those states are Washington, Maine, California, Connecticut, Arizona and Pennsylvania. In spite of the many health benefits of dairy products in their natural organic state, raw milk has been demonized in this country since the 1950's. Once again, the FDA and the USDA are working their political agenda to conceal the truth from the public.

One of the greatest benefits of raw milk is the presence of a unique fatty acid called "conjugated linoleic acid" or CLA. As noted earlier, the proper balance of fatty acids is absolutely essential for total health. CLA is a known cancer-fighter and may help reduce body fat. It is found in organic raw milk but not in the commercial milk available in most stores.

Not surprisingly, the M-Field Signature Matching tests demonstrate that the body responds favorably to the energy of dairy products from organic sources but rejects the energy of commercial dairy products.

Organic Eggs versus Commercial Eggs

There are vast differences between true organic eggs and the commercial eggs offered in the grocery store. Those distinctions are evident as soon they are cracked open. Looking at them side by side, the organic egg has a hard and thick shell, while the commercial egg often has a weak shell that can easily be broken. If the content of each egg is placed onto a flat surface, it is obvious that the commercial egg white is much less viscous, running in many directions, while the organic egg white is thick and stays intact. Looking at the yolk in each egg, the color of the commercial yolk is often a pale yellow, while the color of the organic egg yolk is almost orange.

These obvious visual differences can be explained by the level of nutrition contained in each type of egg. *The Mother Earth News* group does periodic checks on the nutrition levels of commercial eggs versus their organic counterpart. When compared to the U.S. Department of Agriculture (USDA) data on the nutrient value of commercial eggs, eggs from hens raised in a pasture environment contain approximately three times more vitamin E, sixty percent more vitamin A, twice the level of omega-3 fatty acids, seven times more beta carotene, thirty percent less cholesterol and twenty five percent less saturated fat.

We can assume that these differences can be accounted for by the environment and diet of the two types of hens involved in the egg-laying process. Purveyors of propaganda from the commercial egg industry would have us all believe there is no significant difference in the nutritional value. If the visual inspection is not convincing enough, I recommend cooking some up and tasting the difference.

Eggs are one of the healthiest foods in the world. They are even more healthful if they are consumed raw, like I used to do as a child. I would take a raw egg and mix it in the blender with some raw milk and Ovaltine, although I would never consider doing this today with a raw commercial egg because it is well documented that commercial eggs are more likely to carry infectious bacteria than true organic eggs.

In describing "true organic eggs", I am making a distinction between chickens that are fed a vegetarian diet of grains and chickens raised in their natural habitat. Chickens are not vegetarian; they eat worms, grubs, and all sorts of non-vegetarian things. Once again, an egg container claiming that the chicken is fed a vegetarian diet is a marketing campaign. As for the commercial hen's diet, the main ingredients are genetically modified corn, soy and cottonseed. This is true even when the label states that the chickens are *free-range*.

The *free-range* moniker is another marketing ploy. What does free-range mean anyway? The term implies that the chicken is free to roam at will; the truth is something different all together. Often times, these "free-range" chickens are cooped up for all but a few minutes per day. Then, the henhouse doors are thrown open and they are allowed access to a barren lot on the outside, if they desire. Based upon typical chicken behavior, they *do not go outside* because they *have never been outside*, yet the chickens and their eggs are still allowed to be called free-range. In my opinion, this is NOT a free-range hen.

At the local level, the best way to find high quality real organic eggs is to check with your health food store. If they do not carry them in the store, the employees are a good source of knowledge to help you find a trusted local farmer. As expected, the quality of the commercial eggs' *energy signature* is not the same as that of their foraging counterpart.

Nightshades

Part of the routine testing procedure includes screening for sensitivity to the nightshade family of plants. Although the foliage on these plants is considered toxic if eaten, the vegetables themselves are usually not a problem. The reason we test for them during our procedure is that nightshades have been linked to inflammation in a certain percentage of people who are sensitive to alkaloids.

Vegetables within the nightshade family are potatoes, tomatoes, eggplant, sweet peppers, hot peppers, and black pepper. There are other members of the nightshade family, but the ones named here are the common culprits. Nightshades can be a problem for people who are prone to arthritic inflammation. According to an article written by respected author and physician, Jonathan V. Wright, M.D., laboratory tests cannot verify a link (Mercola). However, sensitive people seem to symptomatically improve when these foods are removed from their diet. My personal experience in dealing with arthritic flare-ups in my patients suggests that tomatoes, more than any other nightshade, seem to precipitate inflammation.

Chapter 17

Sources of Autotoxemia #2:
Chemicals and Heavy Metals

*We are living in a world today where lemonade is made
from artificial flavors and furniture polish is made from
real lemons.*

-*Alfred E. Newman*

The subject of chemicals in our environment is a book unto itself. In 1967, the United States Environmental Protection Agency (EPA) launched a program to measure levels of toxicity found in human fat. The EPA did this for a number of years, but the research has since been discontinued. The program was called the National Human Adipose Tissue Survey (NHATS).

The NHATS survey was conducted annually by taking fat samples from surgical patients. The fat was then analyzed, looking for 54 different environment chemical toxins. Recall that the body uses fat for storage of energy and as a place to store toxic chemicals until the body has the means to eliminate them, if ever.

In the NHATS survey, extremely high levels of five chemicals, (one dioxin and four solvents), were found in *every sample* tested! Another nine chemicals, including benzene, toluene, and DDT, were found in over 90% of all samples, while PCBs were found in 83% of all samples. In 76% or more of all samples, a total of 20 toxic compounds were found (Birnbach).

These findings, as shocking as they are, were found more than two decades ago. The number of new chemicals introduced into our environment since that time runs into the thousands. How much longer can we continue to dump chemicals and toxins into the environment and still survive? Even the FDA admits that we are consistently exposed to increasing levels of toxic chemicals, yet they continue to allow this to happen.

The Yakima River in Washington State provides drainage for some of the most fertile farmland in the United States. This lush and bountiful valley is laced with fruit orchards and vineyards. In my youth, our family would travel there in the late summer to purchase fruits and vegetables for home canning. I was shocked to learn in 2009 that the Yakima River was found to be "at risk" from chemicals. During a normal irrigation season, more than 300 tons of sediment contaminated with pesticides and other pollutants enter the river from surrounding farmland. Studies have shown that fish in the lower river have one of the highest concentrations of DDT in the country (Birnbach).

The consumer protection agencies of the federal government seem powerless to protect us. In 1958, Congress passed the Delaney Amendment, which "suggested" that commercial food processors should prove that chemicals were safe for humans, but it was not required. That weak law was eliminated by the "Food Quality Protection Act of 1996". The name implies consumer protection when the reality is just the opposite. In 1950, there were 704 chemical additives in commercially packaged food. In 1984, Ruth Winter's *A Consumer Dictionary of Food Additives* discussed 8,000 additives and the updated version 20 years later covered over 12,000 chemicals (Frost).

The end result of all this toxic build-up in our environment is that we have now gotten to the point where babies are born with a huge toxic load inherited from their mothers. A 2004 study by the Environmental Working Group found that blood samples for newborns contained an average of 287 toxins, including mercury, fire retardants, pesticides and the chemicals from non-stick cookware.

Even with the fast and efficient M-Field energy signature matching technique, it is not possible or practical to attempt to screen for all of the different chemicals we are exposed to each day. As a result, we must be content to screen for a few common toxic chemicals for the purpose of identifying a *nutritional defense* against this chemical onslaught. It is possible to identify the prominent offending chemical using the MFT energy technique. Then, the practitioner can use this information to ramp-up the energy of the M-Field enough to gather more specific information about nutritional solutions for each patient's personal chemical crisis.

Along with the GMO-related glyphosate herbicide and Bt biopesticide, the most common chemicals screened for in the testing procedure are acetates, chlorine, plastic, medication, food preservatives and colorings, and perfume. We could get more detailed and screen for many other chemicals; however the solutions for these toxins would mostly be the same. Using the MFT procedure, the tester identifies the nutritional protocol to support the body's drainage organs to help move these toxic chemicals out.

When patients are informed that the M-Field Signature-Matching Technique has identified the presence of toxic chemical energy in their body, many are shocked and immediately want to know the origin of the offending chemical. I explain that everybody is toxic to varying degrees, thanks to all the chemicals in our environment. Although many of us have heard reports at some point or another about the threat of environmental toxins, most people cope by assuming it does not apply to them. Given the state of our environment, the reality is that we can run but we cannot hide; everybody is "polluted."

The ultimate solution is avoidance. In the *area of avoidance* of chemicals, I make the following recommendations:

1. Avoid drinking your water out of **plastic** containers, especially on hot days. Warm plastic leaches into your water more than cold plastic. Stainless steel water containers work the best for daily use. The best water, if you can find it, is well water from a pristine source. I am fortunate enough to get mine from a well at the base of the Olympic Mountains.

2. Do not assume that health comes from taking **medication**; medication is treatment for disease. It may keep you alive long enough to **regain** your health, but it will not **bring** you health. Only nutrient-dense organic whole food can feed and restore the body.

3. If you are eating "**food products**", you're not eating real food. Products are refined, "enriched" with artificial vitamins, have hydrogenated fat, artificial colorings, and preservatives for long shelf life. Prior to processing, most commercial foods are grown on tainted, lifeless soil.

4. Attempt to purchase the most natural **personal-care products** that you can find.

5. Use natural **cleaners**, such as baking soda, lemon, and vinegar. The internet is a great resource for recipes for non-chemical alternatives.

Mercury

Mercury is the real "heavy" of the heavy metals. When performing the MFT testing Procedure, the most common heavy metal to *attract the interest* of the M-Field is mercury. A well-known neurotoxin, mercury can be found at some level in every person we test. Almost everybody in my generation, and the generation that immediately follows, has been to the dentist and been "gifted" with silver amalgam fillings in their teeth. In the 1990s, 97% of the practicing dentists in the United States used these types of fillings (Mercola).

The only problem is that silver is a minor component in the filling compared to mercury. Amalgam fillings are approximately 50% mercury and 25% silver. These ratios beg the question: why are they called *silver amalgam fillings* instead of what they really are, *mercury amalgam fillings*? Thanks to decades of deceptive efforts by the American Dental Association and our old friends at the FDA, most Americans are unaware of this fact.

In 2008, Seattle news affiliate KIRO reported that Seattle City Light workers were responsible for spilling approximately a half-cup of mercury. The spill was not properly reported and there was a clumsy attempt at clean up that resulted in making the problem worse. In the end, approximately 200 people got involved in the cleanup. There was a lot of publicity around the event, and the hazards of mercury in the environment were discussed publicly for some time.

If the mercury contents of a typical thermometer where to be released into a small lake, that lake would be shut down due to the environmental hazard. Yet much higher levels are readily put into the mouth when a dental patient receives a silver amalgam dental filling. This disconnect is so obvious that I feel a little silly explaining the problem in this much detail.

It is estimated that 75% of Americans are ignorant about the fact that "silver" fillings are really "mercury" fillings. The good news is that the number of dentists in practice today who still use amalgam fillings is down from 97% in the 1990s to approximately 50% now. This has happened with no help from the FDA or the ADA, who still refuse to acknowledge that implanting mercury into someone's mouth is a bad idea.

The FDA and ADA have defended mercury by saying that it is a stable substance once placed into the teeth, despite overwhelming evidence showing mercury to be easily released in the form of vapor each time we eat, brush our teeth or drink hot liquids. For the past 32 years the FDA has refused to issue any public warning about its neurotoxic risk.

It was hoped that the FDA would reconsider this indefensible stance after the World Health Organization called for the phasing out of all amalgam in a 2011 report. That report details the many health consequences of mercury in the body:

> Mercury is highly toxic and harmful to health. Approximately 80% of the inhaled mercury vapor is absorbed in the blood through the lungs, causing damage to the lungs, kidneys and the nervous, digestive, respiratory and immune systems. Health effects from excessive mercury exposure include tremors, impaired vision and hearing, paralysis, insomnia, emotional instability, developmental defects during fetal development, and attention deficit and developmental delays during childhood. (WHO)

Mercury fillings are banned in Norway, Sweden, and Denmark. Canada restricted the use of them in 1996, and in 2001 the Council of Europe called for restrictions and prohibition of them.

Unmoved by all of this, the FDA said that they would issue a statement prior to the end of 2011. A few minutes before the end of the 2011 work year, the agency issued a statement saying that there would be no statement issued. Not now, perhaps not ever.

The drama around the FDA mercury issue is closely monitored by health and consumer advocacy groups. For those who have a keen interest in this subject, I suggest subscribing to the mercola.com website. It is free, and offers timely updates and a great deal more detailed information regarding to the current politics that seem to control the "opinions" of the FDA.

For my part, all I can do is continue to educate my patients about the dangers of mercury and provide individualized mercury detoxification programs to improve their overall health. This service is easy for health practitioners to provide by using the MFT testing procedure to gather the information from the body through the Morphogenic Field.

Lead

In *Sara's Story*, she describes the impact of her undefined, yet severe, gastro-intestinal problems. Recall that most of Sara's symptoms began rapidly improving as soon as we acknowledged the *energy of lead* in her intestinal tract. I distinctly recall her look of simultaneous shock and recognition as I reported the findings of the M-Field Signature Matching Procedure.

As it turned out, Sara had grown up in an environment where she was constantly exposed to lead, but it had never occurred to her that lead toxicity might be the origin of her symptoms. When it was discovered with the MFT energetic testing system, she immediately knew that it was true. At that moment, as she experienced the accuracy of the MFT procedure, she went from skeptic to believer.

Aluminum and Other Metals

Aluminum is another widely recognized neurotoxin. Sources of aluminum in our environment include antiperspirants, antacids, aluminum food containers, and cooking utensils.

Aluminum has been implicated in Alzheimer's disease. Although the cause of Alzheimer's disease (AD) is not known, research indicates that a buildup of aluminum exists in four sites in the brains of patients with AD. To date, there are many different independent lines of competing research that verify this correlation. (Klan)

In our use of the MFT testing procedure, aluminum is the second most common heavy metal energy to present. In this situation, as with all of the Autotoxemia protocols, we recommend both avoidance and detoxification. As stated before, the detoxification component is highly individualized, and depends upon the person's biochemistry. The avoidance component is accomplished by reducing exposure. To that end, we make these recommendations to our patients:

1. Avoid aluminum based antacids, such as Mylanta and Maalox.
2. Avoid foods and beverages that come in aluminum cans.
3. Avoid aluminum cookware. Stainless steel, porcelain, cast iron, or ceramic cookware is better.
4. Avoid antiperspirants. Although this is easier said than done, options include deodorants that do not have aluminum salts, washing under your armpits daily using a gentle anti-bacterial soap, and increasing your intake of chlorophyll by eating more organic green leafy vegetables or by taking organic whole food supplements.

Other heavy metal energies included in our test kits are titanium, iron, and gold. Environmental sources of these metals include titanium-based surgical implants and inorganic iron contained in some low-quality minerals supplements, and for some, even gold content in jewelry.

There are many other possible sources of environmental exposure to heavy metals. The ones mentioned above are the most common so those energies have been included in our test kits. In individual cases, more specific testing may be required to identify offending heavy metals. Hair analysis has also been found to be effective in identifying offensive metals. The MFT testing procedure is quick and makes it easy to energetically screen for heavy metal toxicity. Plus, we offer our patients excellent noninvasive nutritional health-improvement solutions.

Do You Have Toxins?

Every person who lives on planet earth in the 21st Century has some degree of toxicity. Although this may sound oversimplified, it is not. The very fact that the Canadian study demonstrated Bt pesticide toxin presence in 90% of the pregnant women and over 80% of the fetal blood supply suggests that we are ALL toxic to some degree. This is reinforced with the recent discoveries of traces of medication within the polar ice caps, increased mercury levels found in pristine alpine lakes, and the previously stated example of DDT in the Yakima River. Considering the cumulative effects of all of the maternal exposure to chemicals and heavy metals in our current environments, most of us were born toxic.

So the question has become, not "ARE you toxic?", but "HOW toxic ARE you?" Famed nutritional pioneer Dr. Royal Lee described the symptoms of toxicity back in 1935 during a discussion with the Natural Foods Association comparing natural supplements to synthetic imitators:

> The average person gets (symptoms of illness) and goes to the doctor and the doctor cannot find anything that he can recognize. You know, poisons cause us to be sick, but they don't cause fever. Anyone who is real sick, without a fever, suspect a poison. If it is some other form of infection, they are bound to have a fever.

How many of us know someone who is "real sick, without a fever?"

Chapter 18

Immune Challenges and Epigenetic Theory

"Serious illness doesn't bother me for long because I am too inhospitable a host."

~Albert Schweitzer, 1952 Nobel Peace Prize winner

Most people reading this have a basic familiarity with the typical response by the medical system for dealing with immunity. The patients I treat who have immune challenges have usually gone the medical route first, where they have been screened for two basic possibilities: bacterial infection or viral infection.

If the doctor believes the infection is bacterial in nature, an antibiotic will probably be prescribed. If it appears as if the infection is viral in nature, the condition is considered "self-limiting" and no intervention is required. Either way, the medical profession is quite good at handling acute cases of these immune challenges. The people we typically see with obvious immune challenges are the ones who have not responded to classic medical care.

There exists a basic difference in philosophy between traditional American medicine and classic natural healing. To understand this, we must revisit the 19th Century debate about the nature of infectious disease.

Two fine scientists, contemporaries of one another, developed competing theories about the nature of our immune system and its ability to protect us.

Louis Pasteur believed that an external invasion of germs, originally called "animalcules" was the cause of disease. Antoine Bechamp believed that infections were the symptom of an internal dysfunction. He argued that the "morphing" of a cellular unit named a "mycrozyma" was responsible for disease. Bechamp felt that the mycrozymas could *morph*, or adapt, to match the current cellular environment. Likewise, the cellular environment can be subject to continuous change, making this a very practical arrangement. It is rumored that Pasteur, at the time of his death, believed that he had been wrong and that Bechamp's theory was correct.

Although the truth is probably a combination of both theories, the medical community has historically supported Pasteur's thinking. Meanwhile, the natural health care community has a tendency to look at immune issues similarly to Bechamp. Once again, it is the **environment** that we have traditionally focused on to build the total health of the individual. Natural healthcare theory fits perfectly into the current accepted wisdom regarding epigenetics.

If the patient can control their environment, epigenetic science posits that they can control their genetic expression. This applies not only to the present, but also for generations that follow. Part of the epigenetic theory maintains that controlling the environment in one generation manifests in the next generation. For better or for worse, the health of the current generation of young people determines the health of our future generations.

Just as the "primitive people" of Dr. Price's research were adamant about feeding special nutritious foods to the young couples in their child-bearing years, we must also ensure the survival of the species by improving the health of our youth. Our current American diet of processed food and drinks containing high fructose corn syrup, excessive amounts of sugar, nitrates, preservatives, and hydrogenated fats do not contain the building blocks of a strong body.

A lack of proper immunity is just one of the consequences.

The Different Types of Immune Challenge

Scavengers

In MFT, there are labels for the different types of immune challenges, based upon their "mode of operation." Most people are aware of the existence of bacteria, viruses, yeast, mold, fungus and parasites in the human body. The problems caused by an imbalance of these entities are numerous and well documented. However, because MFT does not detect the presence of *actual* parasites but parasite *energy*, these problem-causers are referred to by the role they play in challenging the immune system. In MFT, the bacterial energies are called "the scavengers", because their job is to clean up the dead and dying tissue in the body, and make it disappear. Without pathogenic bacteria in our environment, road kill would be with us forever.

The recurring presence of pathological bacteria imbalance in the body implies that there may be too much food available for the scavengers; in other words, there is too much dead and dying tissue in the body. This is a sign of a poorly nourished body, one that is "starving to death." Rather than piling on the antibiotics, these patients need to be treated for the long term using good nutrient-rich, organic food. For many of them, it probably means a radical lifestyle change if they hope to ever be healthy again.

Replicators

Viral energies are called "the replicators", because of the way viruses reproduce. They takeover a weak cell, begin to replicate, and then spread to other cells. Chronic viral infections are another sign of poor dietary habits that create deficiencies in the nutrients that build strong connective tissue and mucous membranes.

For people who are frequently sick with viruses, the most important nutritional consideration is ingesting sources of whole food vitamin C. Again, it is important to discriminate the source of the vitamin. Ascorbic acid, the synthetic form of vitamin C that is prevalent in processed food, is not the same as whole food vitamin C complex. Vitamin C and its supporting nutrients are not manufactured in the human body; they must be part of the diet. We can only get them through eating real food or taking an organic whole food supplement.

Although there are other factors involved in viral resistance, Vitamin C complex is the most important component. I do not advocate taking massive amounts of vitamin C. If the source of supplementation contains all of the elements and synergist from the Vitamin C *Complex*, much smaller dosing is required.

Proliferators

Microbes that form the yeasts, molds, and fungus families are grouped together into a category called "the proliferators". Although all three of these can be considered separate entities, they have many similarities. They tend to start small and spread out over wider areas, as in the case of athlete's foot or a yeast infection.

Our immune system handles each in a similar way. Approximately 70% of our immunity comes from our intestinal tract. Since our intestinal tracts are under such great stress these days because of the food we put into our bodies, it is not uncommon to develop the condition called *dysbiosis*. In this condition, the normal gut microbes, also called the *flora*, become unbalanced.

In the MFT testing procedure, it is very common for the energy of the proliferators to show up in people who eat too much sugar, too many refined grains or have been treated medically with a round of antibiotics.

MFT solutions aim to rebalance the microbes and establish normal flora in the intestinal tract. Treating the energy of proliferators will restore a healthy balance, while eating traditional foods that have been lacto-fermented will sustain it. Remember, Dr. Weston Price found fermented food in **all** primitive diets he studied.

Detrimentals

The fourth and final group in the immune challenge side of the MFT Blue Kit is my personal favorite. We are uniquely successful in finding and treating these energies using our testing technique. They are abundant, more so than most health care professionals would care to acknowledge. This grouping is the parasite energies, which are called "the detrimentals".

The definition of a parasite is a microbe that lives **in you** or **on you** to its **benefit** and to your **detriment**. In other words, the detrimentals *suck the life out of you*. It is important to note that chiropractors do not treat parasites. However, we do treat "energy". The spine houses the nervous system, and the nervous system is the energy of the body. As an extension of the energy of the nervous system, the human torus energy field, the M-Field, provides information about the body's exact priority at that moment in time. The presence of parasite energies can reduce the size and symmetry of the M-Field very quickly. Without a large M-Field, the patient loses energy for daily living. As a health care provider, it is extremely rewarding to locate these energies, find the right solution for the problem and watch the patient's life-force return to normal over the next few weeks and months, as was the case with Chantea.

It was difficult for me to see Chantea when she first came into my office after living in California for several years. This beautiful, once vibrant and athletic girl had been turned into a shadow of her former-self. After being frustrated by a lack of answers from the medical community for her obvious, wasting condition, she returned to her hometown of Port Angeles in an attempt to regain her health.

Thanks to the MFT Testing Procedure, we were able to identify the energies of parasitic worms in her intestinal tract, her heart and her brain. Thanks to an herbal supplement from MediHerb® called Horsechestnut Complex, we were able to turn the situation around and return Chantea to her vibrant state within three to four months.

For those familiar with herbal therapy, it may come as a surprise to learn of this innovative solution. To our knowledge, horsechestnut has never been used traditionally to treat parasites. However, in MFT, we do not make nutritional or herbal recommendations based solely upon traditional protocols, but rely on the "M-Field Signature Match" to verify our informed hypothesis. 36 years of clinical practice and extensive training in nutrition therapy laid the groundwork for the formation of the MFT suggested protocols, which serve as a starting place for checking possible energy signature matches. But no specific recommendation is ever made to a patient unless the energy signature is a **solid match**.

Early in the development of MFT, Autumn was working with a client who resonated with a Detrimental Energy from the MFT "Blue" Kit. She was unable to find an M-Field Signature Match to quiet the energy of the parasite. When she took out a prototype test kit that we had been using for experimentation, she found the connection between the energy of Horsechestnut Complex and the energy of the detrimental.

To this day, Autumn likes to remind me that I initially questioned her findings. In my defense, I simply stated that Horsechestnut Complex was used for circulatory issues and not for treating parasites. Later that day, as it turned out, I coincidentally ran into this same client who again related the story of how Autumn had discovered that her M-Field was asking for Horsechestnut Complex for parasite energy. The client went on to say that the pain she had experienced in her abdomen for several months was almost instantaneous relieved when she took her first dose of Horsechestnut Complex.

Since Horsechestnut Complex had never been used in this way, I felt that the responsible thing to do would be to document these findings while at the same time informing the client of the unusual nature of the therapy. Within a day or two, Autumn began checking every Detrimental Energy against Horsechestnut complex and found that there was a definite M-Field Signature Match in many of those cases.

It did not take long for the distributor of the Horsechestnut Complex to notice the unusually large amount that we began to order. Their office called our office to question why we were purchasing so much of it. After explaining it to the distributor, Jerry Linnenkohl of Standard Process NW, he felt the need to report this finding to Linda Ryan, N.D., herbal support consultant for Mediherb®. Dr. Ryan made the same acknowledgment to Jerry that I had made to Autumn; she could find no historical record of Horsechestnut being used in this way.

Just to be clear, Horsechestnut Complex had the *energy* needed to match the *energy signature* of Detrimentals. Horsechestnut alone, without the other members of the "complex", did not have the same energy signature and therefore would probably not work therapeutically in these situations. We have tested both, and only Horsechestnut Complex from MediHerb® has been shown to be effective. This is not intended to be a product endorsement, rather a testimony to the precision and accuracy of MFT.

I can't help but wonder what would have happened to Chantea's health over the long-term had we not discovered these parasite energies in her body. She was getting no help from the medical profession after repeated attempts. Part of the problem is that there are relatively few health care professionals who know how to do nutritional healing using energy signature matching. Fortunately, the MFT testing procedure enables practitioners to detect these immune challenge energies and identify how to treat them naturally and effectively.

Sources of the Detrimentals

Most people, after learning that the MFT procedure revealed parasite energy in their body, have some questions. Where do these energies come from? Are the parasites real, and if they are, how do they get into the body? These are great questions. When asked, I refer to a television show on the Animal Planet Channel called "Monsters Inside Me." To these patients, I recommend that they go online and watch live episodes on the web. Even those who have seen the show before need to be reminded that the parasitologist who narrates the series declares on each episode, **"Everybody has them."**

If everybody has them, why are parasites so seldom diagnosed by health care professionals? It may be because traditional medicine in America has a difficult time detecting the presence of a parasite using standard procedures. The most common way to find a parasite with a standard procedure is to do a stool sample. First, this test must be the ordered by the treating physician. Next, a laboratory technician must know what they are **looking for** and recognize what they are **looking at**. If a parasite is found, the treatment must be effective for that specific invader.

This series of events occurs on a somewhat regular basis, but not nearly often enough, especially when considering the level of symptomatic relief so many of our patients receive after implementing the natural remedies their body has asked for.

Parasites are widespread. They are living organisms with reproductive habits, life cycles, and a will to live. We may encounter them in our food, water, or even in the air we breathe. These tiny creatures can easily hide from us, or plant their eggs on some unsuspected surface which we then come into contact with.

Besides living within our bodies and drawing away energy resources, parasites can give off special toxins that weaken surrounding tissues. Just like any other life-form, they consume food and eliminate waste products, which are dumped directly into their host. This increased toxic load can burden an already overloaded detoxification system, resulting in additional symptoms.

Personally, I have had to complete approximately five parasite flushes in my lifetime. I feel fortunate that I recognized and eliminated them before they created any long-term health issues. Based upon my personal experience and that of hundreds of patients, I agree with the narrator of "Monsters Inside Me": everybody has them, and most have no idea. Patients with long-standing detrimental immune challenges may even feel normal, because they no longer understand what normal feels like.

Jim's Story

In 1996 I was working in a wastewater treatment plant. I was replacing a rusty metal part on the influent (raw sewage) line of the plant. When the bolt snapped, my hand hit the rusty metal, cutting through two layers of rubber gloves, cutting my finger to the bone right at its base.

So I cleaned it, let it bleed for a while, then cleaned it with peroxide and bandaged it. I took care of it to make sure there was no apparent sign of infection.

A couple weeks later, I had a low grade fever with a massive headache. So I went to my medical doctor and told him what had happened. He had a whole series of blood work done on me and could find nothing wrong. I kept getting worse. Soon I had no energy. I got tired just walking across the room. I was a very active person. Before this had happened, I would run at lunch just to burn off my extra energy.

My wife Chris made me go back to the medical doctor. He ran another series of tests along with a CT scan and repeated the blood tests. Again, they found nothing wrong. He put me on antibiotics, which made me worse.

By this time, I began seeing Dr. Frank Springob. He had tested me and started me on some nutritional supplements, trying to figure out what was wrong with me. I was getting some relief from what Dr. Frank was doing. On my next visit to the medical doctor, he said he couldn't help me and told me to continue to see Dr. Frank, but to let him know if things got worse. What I didn't tell him was that things were already incredibly bad or I wouldn't have come back to him in the first place.

141

So I continued to see Dr. Frank and over the course of several months, he got me "somewhat" back on track. During the testing procedure that Dr. Frank did back in those days, he found some immune challenge energy readings in my heart and in my brain. He said that the problem was complex and that he could only treat one of these types of problems at a time, so it would be taking a long time to fix this problem. Dr. Frank also told me that because my energy level was so low, it was difficult to get a reading on which nutrients I needed. During this time, I didn't miss one single day of work. But I would have to take a lot of ibuprofen, since my problem made my neck hurt a lot. Ice packs on my neck helped me get through the day. Some days I didn't know if I was going to make it, I felt so bad. I did not want my wife and kids to know, but they knew I was in bad shape.

At my oldest son's football game, (I would rub his head for luck before each game) I walked down the six or seven steps needed to reach him. I felt like I was going to pass out, but I did not want him to know. But he could tell by looking at me. I could see in his face that he thought I might not make it through the game.

It was my worst night and I had to dive deep inside my core to just make it through the game. I don't really remember what happened during that game. Things had gotten worse before they got better. I lost some of my memory. I could not remember anything about wastewater or tap water that I learned in the past three to four years. I could not remember how to do math in my head anymore. I couldn't remember the names of people that I had known for a long time.

I had to relearn a lot of things. I still have a hard time with names. It seemed like each summer, after being exposed to the warm sun, I would have to start all over again. Dr. Frank said that the radiation of the sun, increased free radicals in the body and that created new stresses. The stresses would show up in the "energy" of my kidneys, spleen, heart and liver. Dr. Frank advised that I avoid the sun and other things that I seem to be developing allergies to, such as caffeine and sugar.

When Autumn Smith, NTP began her nutritional therapy practice, I started to see her on a regular basis. She had figured out that if you got people's energy level increased by improving their diet and giving them the right nutritional supplements, you could help them find the real problem. Autumn said that she and Dr. Frank working together had developed a new way of nutritional testing. We were working on both diet and nutrition to get my energy level up. She found other foods that my body didn't want and got me on nutrients for my other issues at that time. Before long, I was doing the best I had in years.

Then in late December 2010, I drove my son back home from San Diego, driving a total of over 2500 miles. When I got home I saw Frank and Autumn each once. After testing me, Dr. Frank said that the long drive had "dropped my kidneys", which he worked back up. Autumn gave me some nutrition for what she said was mercury toxicity due to old fillings in my teeth. She said I needed follow-up treatment but she was going on maternity leave.

One morning soon after, I bent over to feed my cats and I had a muscle spasm in my low back over the area of the kidney. The spasm put me on my back half in and half out of the doorway. I couldn't move for over one-half hour without going into severe spasm and intense pain. I finally crawled back to the refrigerator and got an ice pack.

I went to see Dr. Frank, but when I got out of my chair I went down to my knees with another spasm. I couldn't get up for a while. On my next visit Frank and his wife Linda, who is also a nutritional therapist tested me and figured out what nutrients I needed to help me get through this crisis. As I was leaving I had another spasm in the parking lot. Linda called Dr. Frank to help me to my car.

When Autumn came back to work she began an intense program to work around me and get my energy level backup, though it was slow at first. She continued to work on the nutrients for my heart, kidneys, liver and spleen to get them *healthy again. Apparently, I have had an ongoing problem with mercury. I reported to Autumn that my feet were hurting badly so she started me doing foot baths to move mercury and other toxins out. This helped a lot.*

Within five or six months, Autumn had an old man feeling young again! Although I still have some ongoing problems, this is the best I've felt in almost 20 years. Dr. Frank has developed a great team at the Wellness Center.

Chapter 19

Cell "Blueprints"

"I can predict the success of any construction project by observing how many sets of blueprints are available to the crew. The fewer sets of blueprints, the more problems there will be."

–Matt Springob, commercial electrician

As discussed earlier, there are three items needed for a successful *cellular construction project*: a clean construction site (little or no toxic waste), quality building materials (quality organic whole food), and the cellular blueprints to put it all together. The cellular blueprints are called Protomorphogens™ (PMG's).

To build an ideal cell, not only are these three factors required, but they must be in a *proper balance*. If there is a shortage of building materials, the construction project will be incomplete. As evidenced in the discussion of present day commercially processed food, the next generation faces a very real issue of diminished nutrients. If our children are consuming food which is devoid, we cannot expect their bodies to be resilient. Eating white bread, sugar-charged breakfast cereal, processed lunch meat and genetically modified grains grown on poisoned and lifeless soil will never create an ideal cell, tissue, organ, organ system or organism. It will, however, create a "toxic waste dump" in the body—another barrier to cellular construction.

Imagine a person who has been diligent about eating a high quality, organic whole food diet for several years. They have avoided mercury fillings in their mouth, and have stayed away from trans-fats, high fructose corn syrup, and GMO foods. Then, if they also have sufficient cellular blueprints, they should have everything needed to *complete the project*. The MFT procedure confirms that there are plenty of *sets of blueprints,* in the form of PMG's, hanging around the construction site.

PMG's are found in all living cells. Not only do PMG's serve the purpose of providing cellular blueprints, they also play a role in assisting immunity. An insufficiency of PMG's creates a situation in the body where it cannot efficiently regenerate itself as the cells *turn over* each day. It is estimated one out of every 1000 cells in the body is replaced each day by a healthy new cell, assuming the raw materials and other environmental factors are in place to efficiently create the new cells. This is epigenetics at work.

Fortunately for us, if we don't have enough PMG's of our own, we can procure an ample supply from an *outside source*. There are approximately 23 different types of tissue in the body, each with its own distinct Protomorphogen™. A unique feature of these 23 different types of PMG's is that they are not "species specific". They are "tissue specific", which means we can borrow some from another species when needed. If the body's defenses have been compromised for any reason over a prolonged time frame, our own cells will not have enough available PMG's available for rapid growth and reproduction. Fortunately, it is possible to purchase *PMG supplements.*

PMG's are essential for effective immunity. The Protomorphogen™ provides a cellular defense against the body's own immune system, which will sometimes get *revved-up* when there is an invasion against the body. Following a bacterial, viral, yeast or parasitic attack, the immune system can get excessively *charged up* and actually do damage to healthy tissues if there are insufficient PMG's available.

For this reason, MFT must address *PMG availability* in the nutritional protocols. It is not always necessary to supplement the patient with PMG's, but it is necessary to *evaluate them*. The MFT procedure must ensure sufficient quantities of blueprints are there to complete the healing process as new cells are created.

The primitive peoples studied by Dr. Weston Price all had a routine of ingesting organ meats in some form. Recall the aboriginal people from Canada, who explained to Dr. Price how they cut up the adrenal gland and distributed it evenly among the family members so everybody got a section. Besides the obvious nutritional factor of vitamin C complex available in the adrenal gland, everyone consuming it also got a healthy dose of adrenal PMG's in the bargain.

Some readers may recall occasional family dinners where liver and onions were served. This does not happen on a regular basis in America anymore. One of the reasons is the cattle, which provide the liver, are now consuming a diet which creates so much toxicity that eating the liver is no longer recommended. Again, eating organic liver would provide liver PMG's and many other nutrients that are now hard to come by in a typical American diet.

When I was a child, once or twice a month my mother would serve *beef heart* for dinner. There was an ample supply of heart PMG's in that meal. My grandmother used to eat what she called *sweetbreads*, the thymus gland of the beef, which contains *thymus PMG*. She also enjoyed eating cow brain, a supply of *nervous system PMG's*.

All traditional diets included the eating of organ meats, and the people eating them never lacked for the *cellular blueprints*. Today, PMG's are still vital for total health.

Many decades ago, nutritional pioneer Dr. Royal Lee immersed himself in the study of Protomorphology. He created a process for isolating the PMG from the tissues of healthy farm animals and concentrating them into supplements. To this day, the process he used to isolate and concentrate them has never been duplicated. Dr. Lee, the founder of Standard Process®, made them available to the public in supplement form.

Standard Process® is the only organic whole food nutrition company which makes concentrated PMG supplements available. My clinical experience in dealing with nutrition has led me to conclude that MFT would not be an accurate or viable testing procedure without including patient access to the Standard Process® line of Protomorphogens™ supplements. That said, I must add that my allegiance is not to the Standard Process Company, but to those substances that promote health. If another company produced an equally effective PMG supplement, then I would recommend that one without reservation.

Alexia's Story

I was 38 years old and I felt 80! Chronic knee pain, acute neck pain, multiple miscarriages, an ectopic pregnancy, spotting three weeks before my period, heavy periods, hypothyroidism, anemia, blood sugar imbalances, vertigo that eventually became acute and required hospitalization, frequent night time urination, hair falling out, acute acne, facial hair growth, fragile fingernails, several crowns and root canals, teeth movement, gallbladder removal, acute cravings for sweets, pasta, bread, pie, cookies etc., teeth grinding, weight gain, inability to feel satiated, poor sleep, chronic fatigue, fibroids in my uterus, cervix and breasts, depression, anxiety, high stress levels, low sex drive, problems with rage/anger, memory loss, brain fog …

The list went on and on. So why shouldn't this happen to me? Because I am the daughter of a Chiropractor and the wife of a Chiropractor, a group fitness instructor and, at the time, I was ashamed to admit, that I am a Nutritional Therapist. Even with all my symptoms, I believed that I have lived a pretty holistic life, therefore, I thought, "I should be healthy". The fact is that I was too young to have all those symptoms! My body wasn't supposed to start breaking down at such an early age right?

I went to Endocrinologists, Naturopaths, Dermatologists, Chinese Herbalists, Gynecologists, and an MD. They all gave me something to take or apply topically, but nothing worked. So why couldn't my doctors help me?

This past summer I picked up where I left off 13 years ago. I decided to attend a seminar being offered by Dr. Springob and Autumn. I had previously been exposed to "energy work" from my father so I was open to what they were teaching. My intention was to learn the MFT procedure so that I could use an efficient muscle testing technique to help my clients, but what I hadn't anticipated was how this technique would uncover my own hidden health issues, while at a seminar. As part of the weekend seminar, Dr. Springob and

Autumn test each practitioner. While testing me, the MFT procedure uncovered why I was feeling so miserable all the time. Dr. Springob found mercury in my cervical spine, parasitic activity in my uterus, heart and liver and a severe imbalance of essential fatty acids. Needless to say, I left the course feeling overwhelmed. There was a lot of repair work for me to do in my body.

It is believed, in the holistic health field, that for every year you have had a "symptom" or "condition", that you have one month of "repair work" ahead of you to reach optimum health. Looking back into my childhood, as a little girl, I remember having ring worm a couple of times and at the age of 17, I had a ruptured cyst on my ovary. So that equates to 38 months of healing! Yes, over 3 years of regular and consistent nutritional therapy, dietary changes and physical exercise to repair years and years of malnutrition and parasitic destruction to my body.

Dr. Springob and Autumn have been my mentors for the last several months to help me heal myself. Due to a long commute I consult with them via email. Since starting the protocol in June of 2011 I have made huge changes and strides in my health.

After a month on the prescribed protocols by both Dr. Springob and Autumn, my three year acute neck pain was gone! Unbeknownst to me, the heart parasite was weakening my heart which caused radiating pain up to my neck. My supplement protocols changed weekly for several months. There were days I felt I couldn't get out of bed and others that I had surpluses of energy because my energy was so high! Now my energy is up all the time, I workout three days a week with a trainer, and I am starting to feel younger than my age of 43!

During this time I learned about Genetically Modified Organisms (GMO) and how they destroy the body – so out went any food made from a GMO. I changed to an organic diet, wash all of my fruits and vegetables before consuming, prepare homemade bone broths and use the mineral dense broths in my cooking and as stock for my soups, eat very little grains and minimal refined sugar or processed foods. I stopped using fluoride toothpaste, changed all of my household cleaners to non toxic cleaners that I make from my own kitchen, changed all my make-up and body lotions to holistic products that did not increase my estrogen levels, and I take daily whole food supplements and smoothies that target each of my specific issues. My motto is: "if it's not alive then it can't keep me alive". So I eat REAL now, real food that has life to it. And yes, I eat meat. A lot of it!

The most frustrating thing for me, as someone who works in the health care profession, is that not one of my doctors or "specialists" gave me this information for my system to begin to heal. Not one of them said "let's look for parasites" or "you are estrogen dominant" or "your liver isn't functioning right... and if it's not working...neither are you!"

*Thanks to Dr. Springob and Autumn, I am nine months into my healing and I am a completely different person. I saw my Naturopath today and she dropped my thyroid medication one grain, and said "whatever you are doing keep it up because you look fantastic!" Needless to say, I gave her Dr. Springob's information. It's time that the holistic and medical professions wake up and start treating the **_cause_** of the symptoms, not using drugs to mask them.*

I want to invite you to join me on this journey to true health, a level of health that transforms your body on a cellular level. It will literally change your life! You will never regret the decision!

Alexia Sandifer, NTP

Chapter 20

Special Situations:
Handling the "Diagnosis"

"And we have made of ourselves living cesspools, and driven doctors to invent names for our diseases."

~Plato

Many times new patients and clients will come to our Wellness Center after another provider has given them a "label", or diagnosis, to categorize their symptoms. Usually the diagnosis is the result of extensive medical testing. Often the person who gave them the label was a medical doctor who has been extensively trained in this form of health care. The next step following the *pronouncement* of the diagnosis is the list of *treatment options* for that label. Typically, one of the options includes a cocktail of medications produced by big pharmaceutical companies.

When a patient comes to us under these circumstances, it means they either question the label, don't care for the proposed treatment options, or have already tried the medical recommendations and rejected them due to lack of success. By the time they arrive at our office, they are looking for natural alternatives. They have already been to the "real" doctor; now it is time to try something else.

More often than not, the dialogue goes something like this: "Can you do anything for _____?" (filling in the blank space with the diagnosis). This presents us with an opportunity to explain the premise of natural healing and MFT. Although there is an interest and possibly even a commitment to natural health care alternatives, it takes a very long time to undo years of cultural conditioning. People expect us to work with their diagnoses and treat their diagnoses. In our facility, we never use the term "diagnosis". We don't diagnose anything and we don't treat the diagnosis; we treat *energy*.

The diagnosis comes about after a structured medical review which includes several evaluative tests. What we do in our Wellness Center does not fit the accepted definition of the term "diagnosis." Instead, we refer to the MFT Procedure as an "analysis" of the patient's M-Field. Sometimes it is difficult for patients to convert to our terminology, but we never allow the "D" word to be used in our facility.

The Development of the "Special Situations" Test Kit

The accomplishments of the MFT Basic Test Kits prompted Autumn and I to continue exploring ways to apply the technique to more and more complex health situations. The ideas kept flowing about how to use the *energy gifts* that we had been given to expand patient understanding about the real power of whole food nutrition in supporting chronic health issues. As the method evolved, we came up with a new idea for using our *layering* sequence, borrowing a concept from the realm of homeopathy.

"Nosode" is a homeopathic term that describes an energy signature from an aberrant tissue sample taken from a person who has been diagnosed with a disease. Autumn and I designed a new test kit that included the energy nosodes of some commonly labeled conditions that patients routinely ask about. We reasoned, for example, that we could create a test kit that included the nosodes of common conditions such as "rheumatoid arthritis" or "hepatitis."

Next, using our layering concept, we combined the nosode energy vials with those Morphogenic Protein energies *that would logically fit the labels* that the nosodes represented. An example of this was our "Mental Depression" vial, which is a mixture of the nosode of *Mental Depression* combined energetically with the *Brain Morphogenic Protein*.

We hypothesized that these energy combinations might create the same successful *ramping-up* of the M-Field as we found when we created the MFT Basic Test Kits. Not only was it successful, it was incredibly successful! The combinations amplified the M-Field, making it easier to gather information and identify solutions. We decided to call our new test kit "Special Situations." In this test kit, we have vials for 60 *common medical labels*. Now, when patients come in looking for nutritional solutions for their labels, we can answer the question. We don't have to <u>tell</u> them the answer; we <u>show</u> them the answer.

The Special Situations Procedure

Briefly, here is how the procedure works: The patient comes in and gives us their label. We pull the appropriate vial from the MFT Special Situations Test Kit, and test to make sure that the energy signature of the label matches the M-Field signature of the patient. If it attracts, we assume that the label/diagnosis has been given appropriately. We measure the field *with and without* the appropriate "Special Situations" vial. If the size of the M-Field increases, then the patient will continue to hold the vial while we perform the MFT Basic Procedure.

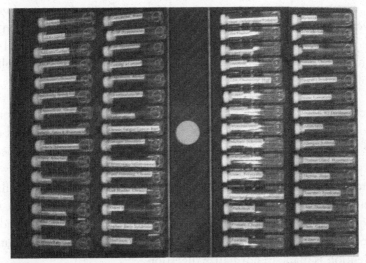

The MFT Special Situations kit contains the energy of many common labels presented by patients. These nosodes are combined with the appropriate Morphogenic Proteins to create an amplified M-Field response.

With the energy signature of the Special Situations vials in the field, the M-Field emits a "ramped- up" signal. Therefore, it gives us more specific information about nutritional solutions for *that specific label* for *that specific person*.

For any given problem there are many potential solutions. The beauty of the MFT Special Situations system is that there's very little guesswork involved in developing the nutritional solution. The protocol that the MFT practitioner develops is an exact match to their patient's "biochemical individuality."

In my years of attending professional nutrition seminars, I was frustrated by many of the protocols designed for a specific condition. These one-size-fits-all programs do not honor the fact that each person is an individual unto themselves. All may have the same label, but their history, body composition, and symptoms are different.

The world of health care tends to be divided into two primary schools of thought: *holistic* and *reductionist*. With holistic thinking, the practitioner understands that one cannot possibly know all of the minute details of each person's body chemistry. It is understood that when you affect one part of the body, you affect all parts of the body, even though you may not completely *understand the physiological connection*. For this reason, the holistic practitioner focuses on the *whole person* from every aspect including nutritional, mechanical and emotional. I have been pleased to witness a trend toward the holistic way of thinking during my career.

Reductionist thinking does not honor the biochemical individuality or the physiological entanglement of all of the organ systems, tissues, and cells of the body. For example, a reductionist practitioner might be inclined to surgically remove a diseased gallbladder, while a holistic practitioner would tend towards recovering the gallbladder. If the gallbladder is eliminated without consideration to the fact that it has a purpose, that patient may subsequently suffer from chronic digestive distress. Without a gallbladder, the body will have difficulty emulsifying fat unless some type of outside intervention is made to normalize digestion.

MFT operates from a holistic position, taking the guesswork out of finding the right nutritional solution to health problems, to ultimately enlarge and balance the M-Field. Using the Special Situations Kit, we are able to get the exact nutritional and herbal solutions needed to help the body battle its label. Information which is specific, accounting for each person's history, genetics, and current bodily resources generates a tailor-made protocol.

Recurring "Themes"

As you read the stories from a few of our patients, you can begin to understand how we got such remarkable results in these complicated cases. The nutritional protocol was an *exact match* for both the patient and the problem. You may have also noticed the *recurring themes* of both heavy metal toxicity and parasite energies. One or both of these problems seem to eventually show up in just about everybody we test using the MFT Special Situations Kit. The development of this kit has opened the door to great new healing possibilities.

Two of our patient stories relate to heavy metal toxicity. In Sara's Story, she had two decades of severe digestive distress that was eventually relieved with a program designed to chelate the heavy metal lead from her system. As she told you in the story, this did not happen overnight.

Purification of the body's tissues is much like cleaning out a paintbrush. Most of us have had this experience. When you start to clean the brush, a lot of paint comes out within the first few minutes. When you think you have it all cleaned out, you set it down to dry, only to come back a few minutes later and find it oozing diluted paint. Even after repeated attempts to wash out the paintbrush, you can find residual paint pigment still embedded in the bristles.

Detoxification of heavy metal such as lead or mercury from the body is similar. Over the years, the heavy metal will seep deep into the tissues and become integrated into the cellular structure. You'll recall our discussion of apoptosis, the normal degeneration, death and then regeneration of the cells of the body. Many of the cells, such as those of the muscle and bone, take years to turn over. Therefore, no matter how accurate you are in picking the proper purification program, it will still take years of commitment to thoroughly purge your body of heavy metals.

Symptomatically, the patient will start feeling better within a few weeks or months. However, if the patient feels as if their problem is solved and stop their specific purification process, they will be extremely disappointed when the symptoms return.

My personal experience in treating such situations has led me to provide pointed education at the onset of the detox procedure. I let patients know early on what to expect regarding how the process will play out over the years. I ask them to commit to the long-term goal of continuing the process once it is initiated to experience lasting improvement from their purification efforts.

Some do, some don't. Many people are resistant to any long-term program. While this is difficult at times, because I know the relief that awaits them, ultimately, I am merely offering an invitation. If I could put it on a greeting card, it would read: "You are cordially invited to improve your health by caring for your body and giving it the nutrition it desires."

In Kathy's Story, you read about the correlation between her label, multiple sclerosis, and our MFT findings. When she came to our Wellness Center looking for natural alternatives, her condition had been slowly deteriorating. Now she reports that her medical doctor cannot understand how her condition has stabilized. The explanation that she is on a constant heavy metal detox protocol for mercury energy in the spinal cord does not resonate with many M.D.s. Some skeptics will remain so, no matter what the evidence shows. This is another example of holistic versus reductionist thinking: they may acknowledge the objective improvement, yet they are sure that heavy metal detox cannot possibly be responsible.

Special "Parasite" Situations

There are a number of nosodes of "autoimmune labels" in the Special Situations kit. These labels represent the most common conditions for which people seek nutritional solutions in our clinic. Rheumatoid arthritis, Graves' disease, Rosacea and Sjogren's Syndrome are all examples.

In these cases, and in many others, adding the appropriate Special Situations vial to the M-Field prior to testing revealed a disproportionate number of parasitic energy responses associated with these labels. As these patterns emerged, I wondered if it could be that many of these autoimmune conditions really began as an unacknowledged parasite? It turns out I am not the first to draw a parallel between these health problems. In his book, "Natural Cures 'They' Don't Want You to Know About", author Kevin Trudeau also suggests that certain types of arthritis can be caused by parasites.

Recently, someone in my extended family was diagnosed with rheumatoid arthritis. His general practitioner made an appointment for him to see one of the top rheumatologists in Seattle, who confirmed the diagnosis. He was given a rather grim prognosis and a prescription of prednisone. When he came to my office to be tested using the MFT procedure, we found the energy of a parasitic worm in his system. We began treating it using two anti-parasitic herbal combinations, one of which was Horsechestnut Complex from MediHerb®.

Within a few days, his pain and level of inflammation was considerably reduced and he returned to work. He is taking about half the level of medication he was prescribed and is extremely motivated to continue the parasitic cleanse, which will continue for several months.

These types of stories are almost daily occurrences in our Wellness Center. It would be logical for people with certain medical training to question the legitimacy of using the nutritional and herbal protocols for the labels that people present to us. Most nutritional and herbal interventions do not have the same validity in terms of research and best-practice endorsements. This is partially due to the fact that no pharmaceutical company stands to profit from their use. Likewise, most medical doctors are simply not trained in the use of natural remedies. After all, there is a reason it's called "Alternative Health Care." The beauty of MFT is that it does not treat the disease, condition, or diagnosis, but treats the *energy* of the label in combination with the *energy* of the person.

The difference may seem subtle, but it is extremely important. Many people who practice nutritional sciences are not allowed to treat a specific diagnosis. Using the Special Situations Kit and the MFT Advanced Procedure, it is now possible to show the patient that many of their labels are best handled nutritionally or herbally. In many of these autoimmune cases, natural symptomatic relief can be accomplished within the law and without specifically treating the working diagnosis.

Each of the patients who agreed to tell their story for this book had one factor in common. Their level of commitment to doing whatever it took to improve their health was incredibly high. Each knew what they wanted to accomplish and were determined to follow it through. Although I, as a practitioner, act as an instrument for their healing, these people really healed themselves! They trusted the M-Field enough to listen to its messages. In my opinion, each of these people is their own hero.

Chapter 21

Inflammation

"Research proves that all disease processes begin with cellular inflammation."

Christiane Northrup, M.D.

The number one cause of inflammatory response in the body, beyond occasional trauma such as bruising or a sprain, is the introduction of abnormal food. The body does not recognize the energy of many of the common foods in our grocery stores, as evidenced by the M-Field response. Fortunately, we have the ability with M-Field Signature Matching to identify deviant foods and avoid them.

In the early decades of the 20th Century, the main antagonists of "food-based" reactive inflammation in the body were sugar and hydrogenated fat. Now, with the introduction of new and unusual food technologies, there are many other sources of reactive inflammation for us to worry about. At the top of this list is genetic engineering, which I and many others consider to be our greatest long-term threat.

About 100 years ago, human bodies were introduced to hydrogenated fat in the form of Crisco. According to the Center for Disease Control, within 10 years of the arrival of this new fat, deaths from coronary artery disease (CAD) had more than doubled. It is now known that hydrogenated/trans fats were responsible for a huge increase in CAD over the next 35 years. At the core of this problem, is the body's natural inflammatory response to this unnatural fat.

As the 20th century continued, the introduction of more refined carbohydrates compounded the problem. Sugar, first in the form of sucrose and later in the form of fructose and high fructose corn syrup, added an additional burden to the body's inflammatory response. Finally, the recent addition of GMO's further compounded the problem. Just as Dr. Northrup noted in the above quote, the systemic inflammation resulting from these foods in the body can lead to more rapid progression of degeneration and disease. With inflammation comes pain and then diseases, including cancer.

Inflammation has an important role in the normal healing response of the body. Proper nutrition promotes proper healing, as is the case with the inflammation that occurs when one sprains an ankle or any other joint in the body. The normal inflammatory response is meant to clean out the damaged tissue and provoke regeneration of new healthy tissue. Once the tissues heal, the inflammatory process is reduced and eventually eliminated as a matter of the course of normal recovery.

Imbalances in the body's fatty acids can prevent this process from taking place normally. When the proper nutrients are not present, the inflammation from an injury can take much longer to heal. To make matters worse, eating large amounts of sugar and hydrogenated fat can cause unintended inflammation in joints that have never been damaged.

For controlling inflammation in the body, the omega oils are absolutely necessary. They are the raw materials for making prostaglandins. There are three prostaglandin reactions in the body that regulate inflammation; two are anti-inflammatory and one pro-inflammatory. The two anti-inflammatory prostaglandins, PG-1 and PG-3, need the omega oils readily available to be produced as needed by the body.

Once these processes are understood, it is easy to see that a proper diet, over time, will create an environment where injuries will heal quickly. By the same token, improper diet, a diet high in refined carbohydrates and adulterated fats is likely to result in a life of inflammatory pain such as swollen tissues, arteriosclerosis, arthritis and perhaps even cancer.

Almost 80 years ago Dr. Weston Price predicted many of the health problems that currently exist in our society based upon the degradation of our food supply. However, even with all of his foresight, not even Dr. Price could have predicted how quickly and thoroughly the mega-food industry would infiltrate our food chain with so many refined food products that lack nutritional value.

It is doubtful that Dr. Price could have foreseen the poisoning of our soil with herbicides and pesticides as it now occurs. The genetic engineering techniques, the patented seeds, and the attempt at a corporate monopolization of our food supply were probably beyond Dr. Price's wildest imaginings. But many of the other issues he warned us about have come true.

All of the problems we face as a society regarding inflammation are the same ones that Dr. Price predicted 80 years ago. Although his dire predictions may have seemed far-fetched at the time, they have exceeded even his expectations. It is unlikely that Dr. Price's research could ever be replicated in present day, as it would require access to a civilization untouched by processed food. In this age of omnipresent commercial food, I am not sure that such a place exists.

Using our energy signature technique, we have tested many foods to determine which foods consistently match the energy signature of the human body. As it turns out, almost any whole organic food is a positive match, which suggests that only organic whole food can be depended upon to nourish the body in the manner necessary for total health.

We have also tested the energy signature of many commercial foods. It is just as predictable that the processed and refined food so readily consumed today do not have the energy signature needed to match the needs of the human body. Commercial and refined foods almost universally fail the test. Additionally, the energy signature of genetically modified foods provokes the same energetic reaction from the body that occurs when common poisons are tested.

Although I will not be so bold as to actually label genetically modified foods as "poison", the muscle response test would. Therefore, the practical application of our technique requires that we reject these foods. GMO's are not something that I would put into my mouth, and although it takes a great deal of effort to avoid them in my diet, I give it the same priority as my avoidance of nuclear waste.

Chapter 22

The Truth About "Synthetic" Supplements

"Be careful of reading health books. You might die of a misprint."

-Mark Twain

Daily, patients at the Wellness Center bring in their regimens of dietary supplements with the intention of analyzing them using the M-Field Signature Matching test. People take the supplements for various reasons, often because of a health related article they read in a popular magazine. The awareness that most food does not provide adequate nutrition is widespread; people know they need something, they just don't know what it is.

There are countless ads on television, in magazines and on the internet which make attractive and fantastic claims that a particular product is the health miracle you've been waiting for. Sometimes I sit in my living room watching these ads, picking them apart, criticizing their content and mocking them for my own amusement. I try not to do this in front of my wife Linda, because she finds it extremely annoying.

I too am annoyed, because I know that many of the statements made in commercials are deceptive half-truths. After all, marketing is about persuading us to buy something. Even the most self-aware, market savvy consumers are affected by advertising. It would not be a multi-billion dollar a year industry if it did not work. The most disturbing aspect of marketing is when words in the commercial script are arranged to imply something that is simply not true. A brief examination of advertising will illustrate this behavior is endemic in the industry.

161

If commercials really go overboard in the deceit department, regulatory agencies may take them to task. An example of this is the recent change made to General Mills' Cheerios campaign. The old ads claimed Cheerios was "heart healthy" and "may lower cholesterol", but they were pulled because those statements are incomplete. The new commercials are slightly closer to the truth when they state that "Cheerios are made from oats, which may help lower cholesterol." Note the subtle difference: it is the OATS which help, not the CHEERIOS.

When my children were in high school, I insisted they take a class called "Marketing," because I wanted them to understand how advertising really worked. While we may not be able to insulate ourselves from the effects of advertising, we can at least develop a critical eye for discerning truth from propaganda. To this day, my children still agree I did the right thing.

Pharmaceutical companies spend an enormous amount of money on efforts to convince people like you and me that we need a drug to make us feel better. A 2008 New York University study reported that in 2004, the industry spent 57.5 billion US dollars promoting their products! Some of those products include synthetic supplements.

A "supplement" by definition is something you take to enhance your already good diet and therefore make it complete. But what if the supplement you are taking is doing just the opposite of what you intend?

The premise of MFT is that if something is not natural, it is synthetic. There are five types of supplements we consider to be "synthetic", meaning the combinations of nutrients in these pills are never found this way in nature. The names given to these five types of vitamin supplements are esters, oxides, crystalline, fractionated and "synthetic". When we test them using the M-Field Signature-Matching test, it turns out the body agrees: synthetic supplements are consistently rejected by the M-Field.

Unless supplements are in a whole food form, they are isolated imitations of the nutrients found in real food, but without the "food" part. These nutritional wanna-be's do have an effect in the body, but the effect is more drug-like than food-like. Isolated nutrients are never found in nature without *synergists* to accompany them. If these "synergists" are not available when you take the supplement, the body then removes them from the tissues where they are stored. This is why synthetic supplements may be effective for a short time, and then stop working. You can actually create new deficiencies in the body by taking the wrong supplements.

A good example is vitamin C. I can always tell when the patient is taking a synthetic vitamin C supplement because the first request of their body during an MF T test is for the "real thing": whole food vitamin C complex. The "complex" refers to the inclusion of the synergists that are necessary to work with the ascorbic acid.

With all of the polished marketing of synthetic supplements, it can be difficult to discern the natural from the synthetic ones. When shopping for supplements, it is a good idea to look for some key words on the product labels before you buy.

There is a type of vitamin C supplement which is advertised using the word "patented". The commercial uses the word *as if being patented is a good thing.* It is not. If a product is patented, it is not natural, since nothing in nature can be patented. Essentially, what the vitamin company is saying is their product is *artificial,* but of course, that word is not effective marketing lingo.

We have seen pharmaceutical companies alter the molecules of natural herbs known to have a therapeutic effect in an attempt to patent a new drug which has the same effect. A good example is the herb Withania, also called Ashwaganda. It has the remarkable ability to support the adrenal gland in a way which tends to elevate the mood of the person taking the herb with few, if any, side effects. The pharmaceutical industry has attempted a patented "drug version" of this herb. In many cases, it has been effective in producing the desired effect. However, similar to most drugs, it also has adverse reactions and unwanted side effects.

Other words to look for as you read the label on your supplement are "oxides" and "esters." Also, if a supplement is synthetic, it will use the word "as" in the ingredients. An example is "Calcium 1000mg 'as' Calcium Carbonate". If it is natural, it will say "from", as in "vitamin C 'from' acerola cherries". This "rule" however, is being violated by certain manufacturers.

A few supplement companies have no problem putting a *small dash of acerola cherry* in with their synthetic ascorbic acid, then labeling it as one of the ingredients. Although literally not a "lie", this practice is still incredibly deceitful, and allows the consumer to believe the product comes from a natural source when in fact it does not.

Another disturbing issue with synthetic vitamins is they could potentially contain many nasty solvents and chemicals. All of these factors can lead to an increased toxic burden within the body in the people who take synthetic supplements. Many people are already overloaded with toxins and don't need to be putting one more item into their mouth that will make matters worse. Especially when they are doing it under the false impression it will improve their health.

Chapter 23

M-Field Energy Signature Matching At Home

"If I have seen further than others, it is by standing upon the shoulders of giants."

-Isaac Newton

Readers who have made it this far through the book will have a disturbing level of awareness about the dangers of the "Standard American Diet" (SAD). The evidence is clear that none of us can rely upon the systems of authority to decide what is best for us, or to protect us from harm. Most likely, you are already committed to taking personal responsibility for your health. With all this in mind, you may be wondering how MFT and M-Field Signature Matching can help *you* navigate among the hazards of the environment, the culture, and the supermarket.

Never fear! In the quest for greater health for yourself, your loved ones, or perhaps your patients, MFT has something to offer everyone. For health care practitioners, there are MFT Basic and MFT Advanced seminars offered several times a year in various parts of the country. Natural health care patrons can encourage their providers to become certified in MFT and bring the technique to their communities. And finally, there are in home applications of MFT that anyone can learn. We believe without reservation that MFT, while a relatively new concept, accesses the innate intelligence that all human beings possess.

From that conviction, my wife Linda recently suggested we expand MFT to include an everyman/everywoman component. She envisioned an MFT Test Kit for in-home use, which would include the energies of whole foods as well as the common food poisons, as defined throughout this book.

Our hope is that people will use the At Home kit to get in touch with their M-Field and learn to listen to it. As individuals are awakened to the communications from their M-Field, they will be empowered to choose the foods which support the primary needs of their bodies at that moment in time. The kits might also guide them to know specifically which foods/substances may be causing a negative reaction in the body at any given time.

This kit is in the research and development stage, and we hope to eventually have it available as part of a new series of seminar designed to teach consumer how to use M-Field Signature Matching in their own homes to test the foods that they intend to consume. More information will be available at the website at www.bugsinmybrain.com.

With or without the At Home kit, there are some procedures that can be performed at home which will develop your skills as a muscle tester, and help you become well-acquainted with your own M-Field. In teaching these procedures, I am attempting to give you a sense of autonomy over your health. I do not wish for anyone to continue eating trans-fats, white sugar, high fructose corn syrup (corn sugar), additives and preservatives, pesticides, herbicides and genetically modified grains <u>without at least asking their body its opinion of these artificial foods</u>.

To use these procedures effectively, you must first understand the "limitations" before you can understand the "potentials". Keep in mind that any energy testing you do at home represents a <u>snapshot in time</u>. What you are testing is the "opinion" of your Morphogenic Field at that single moment. You cannot accurately ask the M-Field what it will want tomorrow or what it wanted yesterday. You can only ask what it wants *right now*. And this information is important enough that it is worth asking about.

Over time, regularly asking for the snapshots, you eventually create a bigger picture of the long-term needs of your body. Done in a consistent way, you get to learn about your body and the best way to care for it nutritionally for the long term. Enough "snapshots" and you have a "movie".

One limitation of using the M-Field Signature Matching at home is that the process is much less *structured* than the professional version of the

MFT procedure. In creating the professional procedure, we combined our knowledge of human physiology, nutrition, and many years of clinical experience to create a reliable testing system which finds the priority of the M-Field. The At Home procedure provides guidance for holistic wellness, but it is not a substitute for the thorough, trained analysis of a qualified professional.

Good, good, good, good vibrations...

Some readers will recall the Beach Boys classic, *Good Vibrations*. While most everyone can relate to that special feeling that goes with being infatuated with a romantic love interest, each individual has different levels of "energy awareness". Many of you will be quite skilled at matching the energy of your food to the energy of your body; others will be quite challenged as they attempt these procedures at home. If you find it difficult, do not give up. If you are persistent in your goal to improve, you will; energy awareness grows each time you attempt a muscle response test.

I know this from my own experience. When Dr. Versendaal first tested me back in the 1980s, he told me I did not have enough "body electricity" to do this type of procedure on my patients. I heard his message, but I was just stubborn enough that I was not going to allow myself to believe it. As a result, I became even more committed to learning and growing my energy skills. Now, in the present, I find myself at the same level he had achieved---teaching an energy technique at professional seminars to natural healers.

The M-Field Signature Matching procedures presented here are an evolution of the muscle testing techniques developed by Dr.'s Versendaal, Klinghardt, and Goodheart. You will find that there are many variations of muscle testing techniques out there, and this is not the final say on energy field work. We are pleased to be a part of an evolving science that will bring greater health, energy awareness, and personal empowerment to anyone who wants to claim it.

There's one more limitation I must address: it is much more difficult to perform these procedures on yourself. They are best performed with the assistance of another person who can actually *test the muscle response* of the individual food energies. If for any reason you feel you cannot trust the results of your at home procedures, I recommend you have the technique performed by a trained professional. A list of MFT certified practitioners is available on the website www.M-Field.info. At the same time, keep working at it. As I stated earlier, the more you practice energy techniques, the more aware you get.

Presented here are three different at-home procedures which use the M-Field Signature Matching Technique. In the first two procedures, a strong muscle response is good and a weak muscle response is bad. When the food you are testing is "in the M-Field", a strong muscle will remain strong if the food "matches" the energy signature of the M-Field. A matching energy means the food attracts to you, which is a good result. If it goes weak, then the M-Field, at that moment in time, is rejecting the energy of that food.

It is important to note that sometimes even good food is rejected by the M-Field. For example, if someone has been on a binge of eating organic carrots and then asks the M-Field if it is attracted to an organic carrot, the answer will probably be "no". Not because there's anything wrong with the carrot; it's just that the M-Field has had enough of them and it is no longer interested in having more. Again, the procedure provides a momentary snapshot.

M-Field Signature Matching In-Home Procedure #1:

This procedure requires two people: the person being tested (for these purposes, we will call them "the consumer") plus another person to do the testing (called "the tester").

A. Before beginning the procedure, the tester must make sure the consumer can hold a strong muscle "lock". To do this, have the consumer hold both arms straight out in front of their body with their hands loosely clasped together.

B. The tester puts gentle downward pressure on the hands, seeing whether or not the person being tested can resist the downward pressure without going weak. (The most important thing to remember is this is NOT a test of strength, as in an arm-wrestling match. It is a test to see if the person can *hold a muscle lock*.)

C. If the consumer cannot hold a "lock" against gentle downward pressure, this test will not be valid for that person. At this point it would be best to try Procedure #2 instead.

D. If the consumer can hold the "lock" against gentle resistance, the next step would be to have them hold the food in question between their outstretched hands.

E. Again, have the tester put a gentle downward pressure on the hands while the food is being held *in the M-Field*.

F. If the muscle lock remains strong, it means that the M-Field finds the energy of this food to be *acceptable for consumption*. (If the M-Field <u>really</u> likes the food, the muscle lock may even become stronger than it was initially.)

G. If the consumer becomes weak when the food is added to the M-Field, the energy signature of the food does not match their energy signature, and they now know they should avoid this food at this time. It is that simple!

One of the tests which I like to do in my office is to take the seeds of genetically modified grains such as corn or soy and compare them to the energy of the seeds of those same foods in an organic form. I perform this test routinely because it is such an effective illustration of the toxic energy of genetically altered food. I believe it is important to demonstrate to every American that genetically modified seeds have a much different energy than organic heritage seeds. I hope everyone who uses the At Home procedure will perform this test as well. If the test is performed correctly, you should find the body's reaction to genetically modified seeds is the same as the body's reaction to any typical poison; the locked muscle immediately goes weak.

This GMO test is an excellent way to get "in touch" with the energy. If you're serious about doing these testing procedures to improve your health by improving your diet, this is a great way to practice. Begin with foods you <u>know</u> are good and should stay strong, and then compare this muscle response to the body's reaction when you introduce the energy of genetically modified seeds. The contrast is so significant that even those with limited energy awareness should be able to feel it.

On a cautionary note: this procedure is designed for the purposes enabling people to match the energy signature of their food with the energy signature of their body. It is not intended to be used in any other manner. There are ways where it could be potentially inaccurate or abused. For example, it would be careless to use this procedure to differentiate edible mushrooms from poisonous mushrooms. There are also situations where it may appear that the energetic response is positive, when in fact *neurogenic switching* has altered the communication from the M-Field (more on that in a moment).

Energetic sensitivity varies from person to person, and in no way should the results of the MFT test outweigh common sense. Please use the M-Field Signature Matching procedure in the way it was intended: to identify foods which are compatible with your energy signature to improve your overall health.

M-Field Signature Matching In-Home Procedure #2:

In this procedure, we will use one of the "Reference Points" that are taught in the MFT Basic Seminar. The Reference Point for this test is located directly underneath the ear lobe on either side. This point represents the vagus nerve, the largest single nerve supply in the human body. The vagus nerve is the parasympathetic nerve supply for the upper part of the body and it comes closest to the surface of the skin at the Reference Point.

This Reference Point is important because the vagus nerve is one of the most central elements of the autonomic nervous system. If this nerve is working correctly, the parasympathetic aspect of the nervous system is balanced against the sympathetic aspect. Generally speaking, the parasympathetic nervous system represents the body's ability to "rest and heal". Conversely, the sympathetic nervous system generally represents the body's ability to "get up and get things done."

In nutritional healing, the energy of the parasympathetic nervous system is the primary focus because of its role in the restoration of the body. When communicating with the M-Field through this procedure, we are asking the body if it is attracted to the energy of the nutrition we are "offering" over this Reference Point. Essentially, the question to the M-Field is, "Do you want this or do you NOT want this?"

Again, this is a two person procedure—one person to do the testing (tester) and one person to be tested (the consumer). Here are the steps of the procedure:

A. Make sure the consumer can lock a single muscle. I like to use the deltoid muscle, which means the person being tested must be able to hold their arm straight out to the side and hold a "lock". As with Procedure #1, the tester would exert a slight downward pressure against the locked muscle. Again, it is not a wrestling match or test of strength. It simply tests the person's ability to hold the muscle "locked".

B. Locate the Vagus Nerve Reference Point (VNRP) under the ear lobe on the opposite side of the muscle you are testing. If you are testing the left deltoid muscle, you'll be using the Right VNRP. If you are testing their right deltoid muscle, you will use the Left VNRP.

C. Take the food you were about to test and "offer it" to the Vagus nerve by holding it up against the appropriate reference point. As you do this, put a slight downward pressure on the strong muscle. If the arm loses its lock, this represents the M-Field "rejecting" the energy of that food.

D. If the test muscle remains strong when the food is presented to the VNRP, then M-Field is not rejecting that food and it is appropriate for it to be consumed, if repeated testing gives the same consistent result.

M-Field Signature Matching In-Home Procedure #3

The two procedures we have discussed thus far work very well when two healthy people are involved in performing them. There is a third option, which is the one to use if you do not have somebody else to assist in the testing. The caveat which goes with this test is that in order for it to be accurate, the person has to be able to pass certain "energetic criteria." This test is only accurate if the person testing him or herself is fairly healthy to begin with and *there is no neurogenic switching present.* The biggest problem with this technique is most people have no idea whether or not they are "switching".

"Neurogenic Switching" was described in *chapter 9, The Effects of Scarring,* and was first introduced by Dr. George Goodheart in the 1960s. It is a type of nervous system confusion which can be caused by chemical or heavy metal toxicity, scarring on the surface of the skin, and food sensitivities or allergies. If any of these factors are present, there's a possibility the nervous system will become confused and then "switch" as a result. When this occurs, the information received from the testing procedure will not be valid. In fact, you can do exactly the right thing and get an opposite result. This happens in approximately 10% of the cases we test.

If you are performing an energy signature test by yourself, you will have no way of knowing whether or not you are switching. You might have to find out the hard way. If you are switching, you won't feel well after eating the food that your M-Field has "approved". If it turns out you are a "switcher", the validity of this testing procedure becomes null and void, and it is time to find a certified MFT practitioner. However, there is a 90% chance you are not a switcher, so let us proceed.

The steps of Procedure #3 are as follows:

A. In an open space, stand and balance yourself. Get in touch with this "balance" in a neutral state.
B. Next, pick up the food you are going to be testing and hold it up against your body. Once again balance yourself.
C. As you hold the food, try to gauge or feel a *shift* in the balance. This may take a few seconds.
D. If you feel your body shift, pulling you backward, this represents an M-Field rejection of that food.
E. If you feel your body shift forward, this represents an M-Field attraction to the food, suggesting it is OK to eat it.

Again if you are going to perform this procedure, make sure you get a lot of "energetic practice" first, so you can be confident of the results.

The Future of MFT

While there are forerunners who have blazed the trail for the rest of us, energy treatment is still a new frontier in health care. The notion of accessing the ancient wisdom of the body is certainly not new, but it is new to many people, and it is not part of contemporary American health care. There is no foundation for it in the current medical establishment.

We believe the Morphogenic Field Technique and M-Field Signature Matching procedures hold promise for application in the other areas, including the fields of chemical dependency, mental health, and even for maximizing athletic performance. This entire endeavor has never stopped being a work-in-progress. Our goal is to get this message and this technique out there and begin developing a body of empirical evidence to create sustainable, affordable, effective health solutions to ultimately create a healthier population and a brighter future for us all.

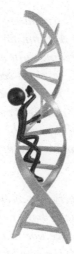

Susan's Story

My name is Susan. I am a cancer survivor.

When Dr. Frank mentioned this book, I wanted to share my amazing experience with Morphogenic Field Technique since finishing my chemo and radiation treatments. Even though finishing treatment was supposed to give me a "happy feeling", I was not "feeling" it.

My body was beat down. I had gained weight. My body was full of scars. Do not interpret this to mean that I was not happy to be alive, because I was. Please understand that cancer is a disease that beats you down both emotionally and physically.

For me it was a question of, "now what?" How do I become me again? While in treatment, I had to focus on just getting through the days and the treatments. However, when it was over, I felt weak. In fact, I was exhausted. It was as though I had a huge impossible health mountain to climb. The people around me felt beat down as well. Plus, they could not understand my sadness. It didn't make sense to anyone but me and it was devastating. I felt I had to climb back to wellness alone.

Now, wellness is my life! A few months after my final radiation treatment, I began seeing Autumn for nutritional coaching and MFT. I started out needing quite a few supplements and changed my eating habits to more vegetables and protein. No more processed foods! I noticed results within one week, including great energy and a new positive outlook on my future. I have lost most of my weight and my strength and clarity of purpose have improved thanks to the testing Autumn has done on me.

Currently I see her once every two weeks. We did go through a couple of parasites that were hard to beat. But each time I just felt better and better. We live in a toxic world but this MFT process is amazing! It is a powerful support for wellness. We will always need the medical community, however MFT allows us to take the "driver's seat" to complete wellness!

I am now healthier than I ever was. I'm doing something I love and each day is a gift. I'm considered a medical miracle to my doctors. I've surpassed any of their expectations as a cancer survivor. If I have any physical complaint, I always check with Autumn and Dr. Frank. I believe in this technique more than any other. I can now look at life from a wellness perspective!

Chapter 24

The End Result

We shall not cease from exploration, and the end of all our exploring will be to arrive where we started and know the place for the first time.

-T.S. Eliot

This book was written for the many people who want to know more about the intricacies of the relationship between the energy and nutrition. What can it do? How does it work? What are its limitations? Can anybody do it? How can it help me? We hope these questions have been answered.

Just like the financial crisis and the federal deficit, our present food path is unsustainable. The degradation of our food supply cannot be ignored. GMO's and their supporting pesticides are approaching *omnipresence* in grocery stores, school cafeterias, airports, restaurants, and farms. How much longer can we continue to experiment on our own citizens with a substance that has historically never been consumed and was never tested for safety? With genetically engineered food, nobody is <u>allowed</u> to test its safety without permission from Monsanto or one of the other corporations that hold the patents!

We no longer have the luxury to wait for government agencies to act; we must act ourselves. Traditional food sources are being contaminated and irrevocably changed. Changes are fine if you are talking about your hairstyle or your toothpaste, but we are talking about genetically altering your food, which appears to have the power to alter your genes as well. It will affect you, then your children and your grandchildren, and all of humanity will live with the consequences.

The Morphogenic Field Technique was a gift to us, and we intend to share its riches by making it available to as many people as possible. MFT initiates an accurate communication, a *quantum conversation,* with the body's energy field. The body is in perpetual pursuit of quality nutrition for its cellular construction project, and the M-Field Signature Matching Procedure lets us make informed decisions about the foods, supplements, herbs, and homeopathic remedies that best support that cause.

If an individual has a specific health challenge, the MFT Procedure can find it. However, treating people who are sick makes little difference if the population as a whole is being poisoned by their food. Remember, the Power that made the body is the Power that heals the body. "The Power" did it all, without Monsanto. Look over that food precipice! If you don't like what you see, do something about it. It is not too late to push ourselves safely away from the "Nutritional Eve of Destruction".

The traditional foods humans have always eaten to stay healthy are <u>no longer readily available</u>. Trusted local sources of organic vegetables, meat from grass-fed and pastured animals and truly free range poultry and eggs can be expensive to buy and not easy to find.

Most people have very busy lives, and consistently preparing nutritious meals becomes difficult given the many other challenges in our society. Most just default to buying prepared foods at the local big box store because it is convenient. For those who have the belief that food is simply another commodity like any other, *cheap* will win. Education is the key to understanding that the quality and nutritional value of food should be the first priority for a healthy life.

Meals prepared from scratch are much different from the commercially prepared foods we have come to depend on today. The ingredients of home-cooked food are known by the person doing the preparation. Do any of us really know exactly what is contained in the packaged foods we assemble from a box? For those who read labels, it can be quite appalling to find out what, besides food, is in that package.

The safest bet when planning one's diet is to buy only food that "grows." This is the common denominator in all real food. For example, everyone knows you have to "grow" carrots. It is possible to go to your garden, stoop down and pull a carrot out of the ground. The same can be said for non-processed meats. High quality meat comes from pastured animals which eat the foods nature intended them to eat. This is how we "grow" the meat.

The bottom line is we need to eat food, not products. Now let's talk about all *the other stuff* for sale at the grocery store. You cannot go to the farm and pick a package of spaghetti. It may originate with ingredients that were once "picked" after they "grew", but there was a lot of processing which had to be done before those ingredients became spaghetti. Some of those steps include milling, stripping, bleaching, and synthetically enriching the flour.

As a child, I ate homemade egg noodles made from scratch by my grandmother. I remember standing around the kitchen table watching the process from start to finish. Everything was made from fresh ingredients and they tasted wonderful! It has been approximately 50 years since this occurred but I still recall it vividly.

I am not naïve enough to think we are ever going back to those times. The world has changed a lot since then, and it is next to impossible to avoid all packaged foods all the time. So the next line of defense for your health is to always read the labels when you buy packaged food. Educate yourself about reading labels. What do all of those big words mean? A 2 second internet search will reveal there are over 50 different names just for sweeteners!

Information on the subject of reading labels is not hard to come by in this age of the internet. If you are not able to research something you encounter on a package, a good rule to go by is, "When in doubt, keep it out!" Beyond that, here are some tips for discerning safe from unsafe foods:

If the ingredients contain soy in any way, shape, or form, assume it has been genetically modified. 93% of the commercial soy is now a GMO.

If the product contains anything related to corn, assume it has been genetically modified. 86% of the commercial corn is now GMO. White corn is currently in non-GMO, so it is reasonable to assume white corn chips, white tortillas and white corn flour have not been genetically altered. However, unless it is organic, it is probably grown on soil laced with pesticides and herbicides.

Some of the most common potentially harmful additives in everyday food are: Sodium Nitrate, BHA, BHT, Propyl gallate, Aspartame, and (my personal nemesis) monosodium glutamate. I can always tell when I have been "MSG'd"; I will have a splitting headache within a couple hours of consuming an MSG food.

MSG is an "excitotoxin", according to Dr. Russell Blaylock, a board-certified neurosurgeon and author of "Excitotoxins: The Taste that Kills". This "flavor-enhancer" overexcites cells to the point of damage or death. It can cause brain damage to varying degrees, even triggering learning disabilities and diseases like Alzheimer's, Parkinson's and Lou Gehrig's, all due to the free glutamic acid. So, always read the labels on packaged food and protect the health of yourself and your family by avoiding these ingredients. The brain you save may be your own.

At times the state of affairs of American agriculture and the standard American diet appear to fall into polarities of good versus evil, as in, "Nature is good; Man-made is evil." The reality is not quite so black and white. Many of the "Frankenfoods" began with good intentions, as an attempt to create more productive crops, less labor for farmers, and more flavorful food with a longer shelf life. Progress is great---but it must honor the traditions of our food supply, which has nourished civilization since its beginnings. You may change the food, but you cannot change the human body. It needs what it needs. If we try to deny that connection, it will be at our own peril. For true health, eat only the foods which have always been here; the foods we now call "organic."

For those who wish to learn more about the history of our evolution into food degradation, an excellent resource is Mary Frost's book entitled "Back to the Basics of Human Health." Frost details many of the battles that have been waged to protect our food supply against those who would defile it for profit. There are many heroes and there are many villains. The reality is, if we are not part of the solution, we are part of the problem.

Action Steps and Contacts

Information is the basis for all future action, but the communication which provides that information must have integrity and be based in fact. The time has come to reveal the truth about the commercial food we eat. The marketing practices which are designed to imply that a perverse food is "healthy" must be confronted. There should be **no food secrets** in America. Every skeleton-in-the-closet must be brought into the light.

In the age of the internet, communication is easy. The electronic media has been a factor in some of our most important recent social changes. Foreign dictators have fallen based upon information released over the internet. It can be used as a tool to truthfully and honestly inform the public; it can also be used to perpetuate a lie. When a uncomplimentary piece of information "goes viral," it is frightening to those who would desire to hide important facts from the public.

The "Pink Slime" controversy is an example of the power of consumer wrath unleashed when a suppressed truth is revealed. The meat industry was caught off-guard by a television news report in March, 2012 that detailed the widespread use of highly processed filler in hamburger. The so-called "pink slime" is derived from bits of meat which are heated, spun to remove the fat, treated with ammonia and then compressed into blocks for mixing into conventional ground beef.

Not to mix metaphors, but the pick slime "muddied the waters" for consumers who expected to know what they were eating in their hamburgers. Within a matter of days, the USDA reacted by stating that beginning in the fall of 2012, the National School Lunch Program will allow individual districts to choose ground beef that did not contain the filler (implying that schools originally had no choice in the matter).

The angry consumer response over pink slime prompted an almost immediate change in USDA policy. As you have read, there are many other questionable policies that must be confronted, and they will be, once the fire of knowledge is lit. When the fire is lit, we need to fan the flames. The problems are pervasive, and lasting change will require a committed, sustained effort.

If you are motivated to become part of the solution, I recommend the following steps:

1. Call and/or write your United States Congressman and Senators and demand Congressional Hearings to explain the lack of empirical evidence demonstrating that GMO foods are safe for consumption. Let them know how they have failed us by allowing

Monsanto and their genetic engineering cohorts to dominate the food supply. For an easy way to do this, go to the Organic Consumer's Association Website at www.organicconsumer.org and compose a letter. We must inundate them with demands to return our FDA and USDA to a state of integrity.

2. For more information on GMO's, go to the website for the Institute for Responsible Technology at www.responsibletechnology.org and learn more about the extent of the damage GMO's have already done to the environment and the food supply.

3. Support the Organic Consumer's Association and the Institute for Responsible Technology, who battle GMO's for you and your families.

4. Support the local organic farmers who are keeping "real" food alive and well. They are the future of food if we are to survive the "Nutritional Eve of Destruction".

5. If you are a health care practitioner wanting more information about MFT, contact Morphogenic Field Technique by e-mail at morphogenic@live.com or visit the professional website at www.m-field.info. There, you will find information regarding MFT Seminars for health care professionals.

6. If you are an individual wishing to take more steps toward a healthier life, visit www.bugsingmybrain.com for information regarding MFT At-Home Seminars. These classes are for everyone to learn M-Field Signature Matching procedures at home. Also available on this site is a list of MFT Practitioners who have the same natural health values that you have.

These simple steps can make a huge difference in your life and the lives of many others. This Earth is our home, this food is our lifeline, and these changes are possible. Political activist Grace Paley once said, "Let us go forth without fear but with the courage and rage to save the world."

Yes, we can save the world. And the world is worth it.

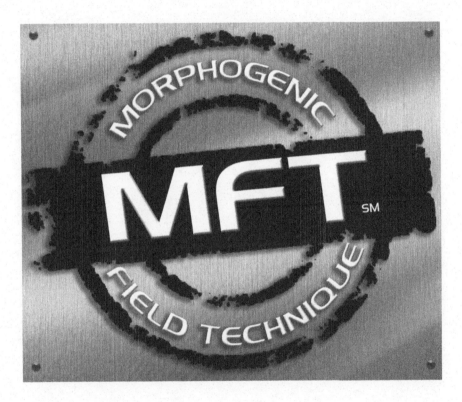

Acknowledgments

From Frank: I would like to first acknowledge all of the patients who have come through the doors of my office in the past four decades. Their goal was to feel better and my goal was to help them. Mostly, it worked; sometimes it did not. The ones who improved made it all worthwhile. The ones who did not improve were the motivating force behind my growth as a health care practitioner and a human being. Thanks to all of you, whatever your role.

I must acknowledge the huge role played by my wife of 34 years, Linda, my partner and office manager for all that time. She endured the long hours, the arguments with the insurance companies, the books that did not balance, the taxes that had to be paid, the frustrations and drama of employees, the endless stream of patient questions regarding their accounts---all this while raising four children who all became productive adults. Along the way, she has risen above the traumatic effects of two serious auto accidents that left her beaten-up and neurologically challenged. In spite of it all, she is still at the office every day with a smile on her face and a kind word for each patient who walks in.

All of the helpful employees and instructors from Standard Process NW gave me the knowledge I need to become a proficient nutritional healer. SPNW President Jerry Linnenkohl is an encyclopedia of nutritional knowledge. My SP representative, Krissy Jutte was immensely helpful in preparing me to give my first MFT Seminar and to this day has always been there, including assistance in editing this book with the help of her mother, Barbara. SPNW Marketing Director Janice Churchill loves MFT and is our most enthusiastic cheerleader; perfect if you are in my position of needing someone who knows to get our message across.

I wish to once again acknowledge the nutritional pioneers who had the foresight to question what was happening to our food such as D.D. Palmer, Weston Price, Royal Lee, Francis Pottenger, and many others.

The oppressive forces of commerce did not want them to reveal what they knew to be true—and they often paid a heavy price to push-back against the power and greed of big agribusiness. Many of them were attacked relentlessly---but they stood their ground and did the battle. We all owe them a debt of gratitude.

There are many people like them still doing the same battle today. People like Jeffery Smith at the Institute for Responsible Technology, and his staff and volunteers. I had the advantage of "M-Field Signature Testing," which made it easy for me to see the problems with the "energy" of genetically modified foods. Jeffery and his people have known it was wrong all along and were willing to stand up to the massive influence of the giant corporations that would poison us for profit.

Then there are "the People". I wish to also acknowledge the crowds that gather when an injustice occurs. Just as always, the unknown faces in the groups are the real catalyst for change. We are seeing it all over the world today—people demanding change in the way their political leaders respond to constituents. Corrupt leaders and corporations who would enrich themselves at the expense of the people are the target of this new political movement. In the end, integrity will win the day. It is "the People" who will see to it.

I wish to thank the patients and clients who assisted me by telling their stories. I present these to show what is possible with the right natural interventions and organic whole food---we have a truly natural energetic procedure that works like no other!

Thank you to Ashley Lynn Smith for her assistance in documentation gathering, which smoothed my writing "process".

Special thanks to my longtime friend, Sydney Upham Soelter. Sydney is a licensed mental health counselor practicing in Port Angeles. She is a true believer in natural health care and likes to help people tell their stories. Her offer to do a "read-through" turned into a "write-through" and the book is so much better for her efforts.

And finally, I must acknowledge Autumn Renee Smith, NTP. She provided the original spark that began the MFT Journey. Her first passion is her young family, which keeps her very busy. But she has found the time to co-create the MFT Procedures and also co-instruct at our professional seminars. MFT exists today, thanks to Autumn.

Frank Springob, D.C. July 2012

From Sydney: Thanks to Clint, Elliott and Hudson for their love and begrudging acceptance of the family time forsaken for this project. Also, thanks to Dad for your open mind, critical thinking, and encouragement. For Mom, thanks for everything…it's too much to list, but especially for your passion for traditional foods and natural health and your unwavering support and interest in everything I do. And finally, thanks to Frank Springob, my mentor and friend who followed his heart in writing this book and trusted me to understand and render his message.

Sydney Upham Soelter, M.A. July 2012

Endnotes

Aronson, Marc and Budhos, Marina, 2010, Sugar Changed the World: A Story of Magic, Spice, Slavery, Freedom, and Science. Houghton, Mifflin, Harcourt, Boston.

Benoliel, Doug, Northwest Foraging, The Classic Guide to Edible Plants of the Pacific Northwest, 2011, Skipstone Publishing, Seattle.

Birnbach, Jeanette and George, 21st Century Clinical Nutrition Seminar Notes, April 4, 2009

Blaylock, Russell L., 1998, Excitotoxins, the Taste That Kills, Health Press, Santa Fe, NM

Braden, Gregg, 2007, The Divine Matrix, Bridging Time, Space, Miracles, and Belief, Hay House, Inc., Carlsbad, CA

Frost, Mary, M.A., 2007, Back to the Basics of Human health, Avoiding the fads, trends and bold-faced lies, Expansive Health Awareness, Inc,

Gagnon M-A, Lexchin J (2008) The Cost of Pushing Pills: A New Estimate of Pharmaceutical Promotion Expenditures in the United States. PLoS Med 5(1):

Gunther, Erna, 1945, Ethnobotany of Western Washington, The Knowledge and Use of Indigenous Plants By Native Americans, University of Washington Press, Seattle, WA

Kimbrell, Andrew, 2007, Your Right To Know, Genetic Engineering and the Secret Changes in Your Food, Center for Food Safety, Washington, D.C.

KIRO television website, www.kirotv.com

Klan, Ayesha, 2008, Science Liaison Officer, Alzheimer's Society

Klinghardt Academy of the Healing Arts and Neurobiology, Official Website, www.klinghardtacademy.com, 12/10/10

Lee, Royal, D.D.S, 1949, An Introduction to Applied Protomorphology, International Foundation for Nutrition and Health, San Diego, CA

Lee, Royal, D.D.S, et al, 2009, Clinical Reference Guide, Revised Edition, International Foundation for Nutrition and Health, San Diego, CA

Lee, Royal, D.D.S. 1949, 2010 The Product Bulletins, Sixth Edition, International Foundation for Nutrition and Health, San Diego, CA

Lipton, Bruce H.,Ph.D. 2005, 2008, The Biology of Belief, Unleashing the Power of Consciousness, Matter and Miracles, Hay House, Inc. Carlsbad, CA

Mercola.com website, www.mercola.com

Moerman, David E., 1998, Native American Ethnobotany, Timber Press, Inc. Portland, OR

Mother Earth News, Ogden Publications, Inc. Topeka, KS, www.motherearthnews.com.

National Academy of Sciences, www.sciencedaily.com, Aug. 17, 2009

Pollan, Michael. 2006, The Omnivore's Dilema, A Natural History of Four Meals, Penguin Books, New York, NY

Powell, Lisa M., PhD, et al, 2007 "Nutritional Content of Television Food Advertisements Seen by Children and Adolescents in the United States", Pediatrics, Official Journal of the American Academy of Pediatrics.

Price-Pottenger Nutrition Foundation website, www.ppnf.org

Price, Weston A., D.D.S. 1939, 2008 Nutrition and Physical Degeneration, 8th Edition. Price-Pottenger Nutrition Foundation, Inc. La Mesa, CA

Smith, Jeffery M., 2007, Genetic Roulette, The Documented Health Risks of Genetically Engineered Foods, Yes! Books, Fairfield, IA

Smith, Jeffery M., 2003, Seeds of Deception, Exposing Industry and Government Lies About the Safety of the Genetically Engineered Foods You Are Eating, Yes! Books, Fairfield, IA

Trudeau, Kevin, 2004, Natural Cures "They" Don't Want You to Know About, Alliance Publishing Group, Inc., Elk Grove Village, Il.

United States Environmental Protection Agency website, www.epa.gov

United States Department of Agriculture website

Versendaal-Hoezee, Dawn and Versendaal, D.A., D.C., 1993, Contact Reflex Analysis and Designed Clinical Nutrition, House Marketing

Walther, David S. D.C., 1988, 2000, Applied Kinesiology Synopsis, Second Edition, Systems DC

Weston A. Price Foundation website, www.westonaprice.org.

WHO, 2011, World Health Organization, Public Health and Environment, www.who.int

Wray, Jacilee, et al, 2002, Native Peoples of the Olympic Peninsula, Who We Are, University of Oklahoma Press, Norman, OK

Glossary of M-Field Terminology

Attraction: When the "test muscle" remains strong during a muscle response test. This occurs as an object, such as a food or a virtual energy vial, is brought into the M-Field or over a Reference Point. There are two types of attraction—to the M-Field (which implies "interest") or to the Parasympathetic/Vagus Nerve/Fatty Acid Reference Point (which implies "want or need").

Autotoxemia: Our term for a condition where an unwanted "energy" has entered the body such as a chemical, heavy metal, or sensitive/allergic food.

Commercial Food: An adulterated food which has been refined, processed or otherwise "acted-upon" in such a way that it no longer has the "energy" of organic whole food.

Cellular Construction Project: The name we have given to the process of building of the healthy new cells needed by the body every day to maintain and regenerate itself. The three parts of the project include the "blueprints", (Protomorphogens™) the raw materials (nutrients), and a clean construction site (no toxins).

Detrimentals: Our term for the energy of parasites. It is based upon their mode-of-operation, parasites can live in or on a host for the *benefit* of the parasite but to the *detriment* of the host.

Drainage Remedy: A natural remedy that has the effect of prompting the body to release pend-up toxicity by supporting the organs of drainage in the body such as the liver, lymphatics, bowel, kidneys and skin.

Energy Signature: The unique resonance or "field" emitted by all objects in the universe. In our procedures, we do M-Field Signature Matching(SM) to find energy signatures of food that is compatible with a person's own unique energy.

Epigenetics: The relatively recent science that acknowledges that genes of an organism will "express" based upon factors in the environment of that organism—such as food, toxins, emotional stress. Therefore, it gives us a measure of control over our genes if we control our environment.

Frankenfood: A common term for genetically modified foods, since they are not the food of nature but those created by man.

Genetics: The science that acknowledges that our genes play a role in who we are, what we become and which tendencies can manifest throughout our lives. We know that 2% of diseases are genetic and 98% are epigenetic. We cannot control the 2%, but environment plays a role in the 98%.

Genetically Modified Food/GM/GMO: Also known as "Frankenfoods", these are foods conceived and created by man through genetic manipulation. In MFT, we do not consider these to be *real* foods since our M-Field Signature Matching procedure universally "rejects" their energy signature.

Gravitational Physics: The physical science that relates to the "scale" of objects the size of the sun and the planets.

Holistic: The school of thought in natural health care that acknowledges that the whole organism is inter-related to all of its parts including organs and cells. You cannot affect *any part* of the organism without affecting *all of the parts*.

Matched Resonance/Energy Signature: This occurs when the energy signature of one object "attracts" to the energy signature of another object, based upon the outcome of a muscle response test.

M-Field Signature Matchingsm: The name for our classes which teach the procedure we use to find appropriate foods that nourish the body and to also isolate artificial foods or toxins that can be detrimental to health and healing.

Mismatched Resonance: The opposite of "Matched Resonance". This occurs when the energy signature of one object "rejects" the energy signature of another object, based upon the outcome of a muscle response test.

Modified Muscle Response Testing/MMRT: The type of muscle response testing primarily used during the MFT Testing Procedure to find matched and mismatched energy signatures. Since most MFT Testing is done "in-the-field"/"off-the-body", we use MMRT for this purpose.

Morphogenic Field Technique®/MFT: The name given to the professional seminars we teach to practitioners of natural health care. The technique is designed to quickly, easily and accurately develop nutritional protocols that exactly match the energy signature of the patient's energy field. The goal of the procedure is the expansion of the M-Field, which represents the patient's energy output. More energy output represents a higher level of health.

MFT In-Home: Still in development as this is being written, this procedure is being created to empower the non-practitioner to make good decisions regarding their food. It does not replace the need for professional support in handling health issues, but you can use it each day to decide which foods your body desires and what foods to avoid as you support optimum nutritional health.

Morphogenic Field/M-Field: The name we have given to the body's torus energy field used for the purpose of feeding proper nutrition to the cells. It is based upon the concept of morphogenesis, described by Dr. Royal Lee in his groundbreaking research titled "Protomorphology, The Principles of Cell Auto-Regulation".

Muscle Lock: This describes the ability of a patient being tested to hold a muscle in a "locked" position while performing a muscle response test. If a "locked muscle" becomes weak during testing, it reveals information that can be interpreted by the practitioner.

Muscle Response Testing/MRT: The name given to a muscle testing procedure where the person being tested suddenly becomes weak when a previously locked muscle is being tested. The loss of the lock is precipitated by the introduction of an outside energy. The sudden weakness/loss of lock is called the "muscle response".

Newtonian Physics: The science of the physical nature of objects of a "scale" the size of objects we deal with in everyday life, such as people, buildings and vehicles.

Organic Food: Foods that have not been altered by man and grown on soil that is free of chemicals.

Proliforators: The name we use in MFT to describe energies of molds, yeast and fungus. The name is based upon their mode-of-operation as they grow and spread.

Protomorphogen™: The "cellular blueprint", which is an integral part of our testing procedure. The "cellular construction project" requires the presence of the blueprints necessary to build a healthy cell.

Quantum Conversation: The nickname we have given to the MFT Testing Procedure as we use it to communicate with the body based upon energy concepts.

Quantum Physics: The science of physics as it related to the "scale" of molecules, atoms and subatomic particles. This is the physics of the physiology of the body at the cellular level.

Reductionism: This term represent the thinking that physiology can and should be manipulated by adding chemicals to the body from the outside. This is the basis of traditional pharmacy. It is a linear concept that does not fully appreciate the quantum nature of physiology.

Rejection: This is our term for the action created by a mismatched energy signature when presented to the M-Field.

Replicators: The MFT terminology for the energy of viruses. It is based upon the viral mode-of-operation where a living cell is invaded and the virus will replicate to propagate.

Scavengers: The MFT term used to describe the energy of bacteria. It is based upon the bacteria mode-of-operation where dead and dying cells are scavenged by the microbe during apoptosis.

Virtual Energy Vials: The vials used during the MFT Testing Procedure that represent the energy of a "real object" in a digital form, much like a DVD is a digital form of a "real performance".